CHILD NO MORE

The Happy Hooker (ReganBooks 2002)

Letters to the Happy Hooker

Xaviera!

The Best Part of a Man

Xaviera's Supersex

Xaviera Goes Wild!

Xaviera Meets Marilyn Chambers (with Marilyn Chambers)

Knights in the Garden of Spain

Xaviera's Magic Mushrooms

Madame l'Ambassadrice

The Inner Circle

Lucinda, My Lovely

Lucinda: Hot Nights on Xanthos

Erotic Enterprises Inc.

Fiesta of the Flesh

Happily Hooked (with John Drummond)

Yours Fatally!

The Kiss of the Serpent

Prisoner of the Firebird

Let's Get Moving (with John Drummond)

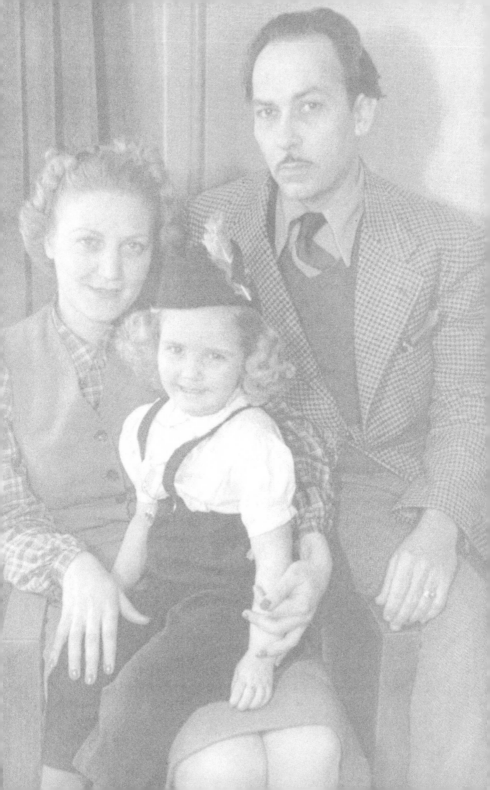

XAVIERA HOLLANDER

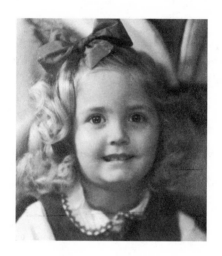

CHILD NO MORE

A MEMOIR

Regan Books *An Imprint of* HarperCollins*Publishers*

HarperCollins books may be purchased for educational,
business, or sales promotional use. For information please write:
Special Markets Department, HarperCollins Publishers Inc.,
10 East 53rd Street, New York, NY 10022.

FIRST EDITION

Designed by Kate Nichols

Printed on acid-free paper

Library of Congress Cataloging-in-Publication Data

Hollander, Xaviera.
    Child no more : a memoir / Xaviera Hollander.—1st ed.
        p.   cm.
    ISBN 0-06-001417-2 (HC : alk. paper)
    1. Hollander, Xaviera—childhood and youth.
    2. Prostitutes—United States—Biography.   I. Title.

HQ144 .H637 2002
302.23'092—dc21   2002022149

02 03 04 05 06 ❖/RRD 10 9 8 7 6 5 4 3 2 1

I DEDICATE THIS BOOK TO

THE MEMORY OF GERMAINE AND MICK,

THE TWO COURAGEOUS PEOPLE WHO WERE

MY LOVING PARENTS.

AND YET

IT IS ALSO AN ODE TO MY MOTHER.

When you are a mother, you are never really alone

in your thoughts . . .

A mother always has to think twice, once for herself

and once for her child.

—SOPHIA LOREN

Contents

CHILD NO MORE

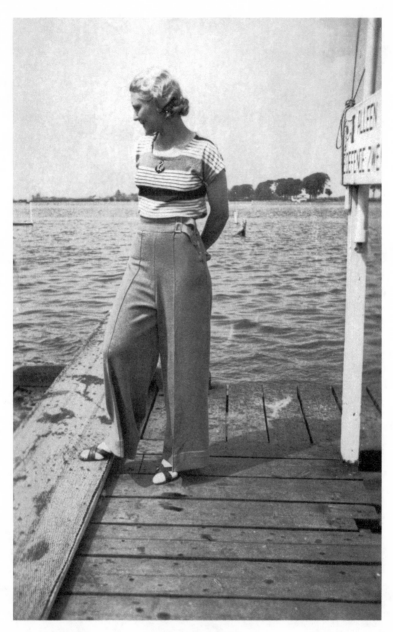

Germaine, 1938

Prologue

DAY ONE. *Tuesday afternoon, July 6, 1999*

I remember the moment I received the phone call from the head nurse. It was seven o'clock in the evening.

"Your mother is in critical condition. You'd better come quickly."

I felt numb all over, and my legs seemed turned to lead. When I tried to move, it was as if some force were holding me back. Even to step into my car and turn the ignition key was an effort. I found that my arms were covered with goose bumps and I was icy cold, although the sun was beating down and it was hot as a furnace. I rammed my foot hard down, breaking every speed limit, but it seemed as if some other person had taken over the steering wheel. This was the spookiest thing I had ever experienced, but more was to come.

I had the impression that my father, who had died long before, was beside me, whispering into my ear for me to control my panic.

"Slow down. You want to help Momma? Then get to the hospital alive."

I sensed his presence, assuring me that this sort of experience can happen when two people are really close. It was as though I were enveloped by a kind of protective cape, yet at the same time it seemed to be the cape of death. My throat was dry. I was choking. And at that moment my only burning desire was that I should die in my mother's place.

I don't remember actually arriving at the hospital and running into the elevator, but suddenly I was with her, alone in a room, and I understood that this was what the nurses referred to as the death chamber. The final chapter was being written in the book of her life, yet she was still conscious, though pale and tired, a blue-and-white-striped washcloth drenched in icy water on her forehead. She was surrounded by a team of doctors.

A young blond doctor who seemed to be in charge bent over her and bellowed:

"Mrs. de Vries? Mrs. de Vries, can you hear me?"

He could have been heard a couple of wards away. She turned her head away. "Mrs. de Vries, your daughter is here. Can you please answer a few questions?"

She nodded feebly.

"Are you sad, Mrs. de Vries?"

She shrugged her frail shoulders and said nothing.

"Mrs. de Vries, do you want to die?" he shouted.

I begged him to stop yelling; after all, she was not actually deaf.

In a soft, clear voice, she replied, "Yes, I want to die. The sooner the better."

I looked at the doctor and pleaded, "Please, now that you have heard that she does not want to live longer, can you do something about it?"

The doctor straightened his back and looked hard into my eyes.

"No, madam. We are not allowed to practice euthanasia, not

even if she had signed all the consent forms." His voice was harsh and grating. "St. Lucas is a Catholic hospital; we are not permitted to help patients end their lives prematurely. The most we can do is to stop all life support: no more food, no more medications except painkillers, and no more liquids. I promise we won't even administer a liquid drip. So she will dry out spontaneously; she will be completely dehydrated within two to three days."

My mother understood every word and looked horrified.

"We stopped her intestinal bleeding a few days ago. In fact, your mother is not ill at the moment. She is quite anemic from losing so much blood, but if she had any willpower she could actually go home and get better there. She just has not got the will to go on living." He shouted in her ear. "Isn't that right, Mrs. de Vries?" She gave him a mean look.

A nurse interrupted. "I am sorry, doctor, but look at the patient's condition. Her weight is down to forty-five kilos. Surely you wouldn't want to send her home in that state, would you?"

I nodded and pleaded with him. "Please, be kind to her. And whatever you do, don't send her home at this stage."

He gave a short-tempered nod, looked at his watch, scribbled a few words in his notepad, took a brief check of her blood pressure and heart, and he and his entourage swept out of the room without even saying good-bye.

By now it was around eight, visiting hours were over, and ward 7A of St. Lucas Hospital was in complete silence. I switched off the big lights, leaving just the light above the washbasin, and moved my chair close to my mother's bed. She was dozing; in her hand she clutched a brand-new handkerchief Dia and I had given her. I sprinkled it and her sheets with 4711 eau de cologne, something she and her mother before her had enjoyed from childhood.

I looked down at her gaunt face, her eyes dark and sunken, and refreshed the washcloth for her. She woke up for a few moments and sighed.

"Oh, I am so glad you are here. Please don't leave me anymore."

"No, Mom," I cried, collapsing against her feeble chest. "I will never leave you again. I'll sit with you until the end."

My mother's life companion, Hetty, had also been with her for the last few hours. Now she took my mother's hand, kissed it, and said good-bye, relieved that I would look after her for the rest of the night.

I had brought a big bag of magazines and newspapers I had not had time to read, and intended to settle down next to my mom. Suddenly, something told me to grab a pen and my notebook and start writing. It had been twelve years since my last book, but now I was inspired to commit to paper every moment of this experience. For four hours I sat there, writing by hand (something I had long since left behind in favor of the computer). It was an enormous relief.

Around midnight, I was very tired. Usually I am wide awake at that hour, but here in the quiet surroundings of the hospital it felt good to try and catch some sleep. I felt utterly worn out, so I climbed into a bed that had been brought for me and placed beside my mother's. I barely slept, waking every half hour to have a good look at my mother, placing my ear against her chest to make sure she was still breathing.

I woke suddenly at five o'clock, unsure for a moment where I was, then got up and drove home. I was struck by the color of the sky, serene in pinks and purples. Well aware this time that I was behind the wheel, I did not rush, enjoying the quietness on the road. When I arrived at my own house my dogs greeted me excitedly, and I found notes everywhere from the people who live with me. I took a quick shower and checked my E-mail, confident that my mom would hang on to life for at least another day or two. But already at half past six I felt restless, worried that she might awake and fret at not finding me next to her.

DAY TWO. *Wednesday, July 7, 1999*

Today was not such a good day: Mom now barely spoke. I had brought with me a copy of a printed booklet I had compiled, a collection of my mom's favorite German and Dutch poems about death, along with three pages I had written as my own offering. The cover was a tender picture of my mom and me during our happy days in Spain ten years before. Christopher, the sweet Singaporean houseboy who lives with us, had neatly bound them with a purple ribbon. The booklet was the idea of an artistic young lesbian friend of mine named Pauline; she spent two days on its layout and printing, creating a lovely memorial for my mother.

Its production was perfectly timed: I read my farewell text to her, and a few tears journeyed down her cheeks. Gently taking my hands, she whispered, "You really do love me, don't you?"

"But of course, Mammi." I tried to smile through my tears. "Why do you ask?"

"Because you did a terrific job preparing all this. Now all I want is to leave you as soon as possible. I just want to go—I am so tired."

"Mom, remember what you used to say? 'It takes as long as it takes.' Be patient; you will soon be there."

During the day, whenever she gestured (and against doctors' orders), I gave her a few drops of water from a plastic cup, and even a few tiny spoonfuls of vanilla ice cream. When she wanted no more, I finished the rest.

She gave me a look. "Darling, please don't eat so much," she murmured.

"Mammi, stop worrying about my weight. I'm a big girl now. Please relax and let's make you as comfortable as possible." Then she dozed off again, and I lay down for an hour's catnap. In the quiet hospital, memories from my youth flooded back.

At about eleven, two very kind nurses washed her. I was shocked by the condition of her body. A few days before, I had massaged her with chamomile cream from head to toe. I can still remember the feel of the texture of her dry skin, and how it came to life under my fingers as I gently applied the cream to her belly, her thighs, and her hands, and then a different cream to her face. I had cleaned her hair with some alcohol—she was too weak for shampoo—and cleaned, filed, and polished her nails.

In the afternoon, I ate the most insipid slop of hospital food I had ever been served. Her body was by now so desiccated that she could hardly speak a word, and I moistened her lips with some lemon water and brushed her teeth.

Time passed. Around four, we had a visitor. Yvonne had been helping my mother and Hetty clean their house for the past twenty years. She was a kind woman with a pleasant round face who considered my mom as a second mother. (Her own mother, now senile, had been unable to recognize her for eight years.) Although she was shocked by my mom's sudden deterioration, Yvonne remained composed until she was out in the hall, then burst into tears.

My mom, who had grown quite fond of my lover, Dia, had asked her to bring a bottle of white wine; she had dreamed of just one last glass of good wine, but alcohol had been taboo in her house in recent years. Now that she was safely hospital-bound, though, my mom had once again become her own boss, if only for a few fleeting moments, and she was like a naughty child as we made our final toast: I with water; she with her watered wine in a plastic cup.

Yvonne downed two glasses, unwatered, but my mother choked as hers went down. Swallowing water had become increasingly difficult for her; now she looked helpless and confused, and her mouth was so dry that her words were difficult to understand. By this time she could barely speak, and we were forced to communicate through signs: the simple fluttering of her eyelashes, the tiny movements of her head.

After Yvonne left, my mother pointed at the table near her bed and whispered one word: *mandarin*. I peeled the mandarin orange, took a segment, and slowly fed her the juice. She eagerly tried to suck the freshness and flavor of the piece of fruit. Gently and elegantly she returned a fragment of pulp, which I removed from her pouting lips. I fed her four more pieces. I have never studied a *mandarin* as I did that afternoon, and I shall never again eat one without thinking of my mother and the way I fed her that last time. Every little sliver of the fruit will come to my mind. *Mandarin:* it was practically the last word I was to hear from her mouth.

She dozed for most of the day, and Hetty and I did a lot of crying. Each hour she looked more exhausted, more wasted, but there was still life within her. Hetty left around nine, and again I was alone, staring into my mom's face for hours. Once again I wrote to pass the time, and I had written thirty pages before falling asleep around midnight, my hand aching with writer's cramp.

It was four in the morning when I drove home, and followed the same ritual as the night before.

DAY THREE. *Thursday, July 8, 1999*

I was back in the hospital by seven. A few hours later, my cousin Harold arrived from Düsseldorf. He was shocked—he hadn't seen his aunt for a few months—but his face was expressionless. Together we sat by her bed for hours, stroking her tousled hair and caressing her chilling body now and then, but she would feebly push our hands away. Her eyes were closed; she responded to us with tiny squeezes of her hand.

When Dia and Hetty showed up, we had lunch and sat talking quietly in the waiting room. But we were too gloomy to have much appetite. Dia soon left; she had some work to do but promised to be back in the evening. Hetty took Harold home for a short siesta.

I closed the door to the corridor. It was a very quiet afternoon; and heat hung heavy in the air. I moved my bed into a corner of the room where I had a good view of my mother. She had opened her eyes only briefly when Harold and I sat next to her. Her eyes were tired and dull; she was breathing irregularly, and occasionally wheezing.

At one point she had opened her eyes, trying to focus on each of us as if for the very last time. Then she glanced at where I had left my little appointment book open on my bed, next to my over-full handbag. The apparent disorder seemed to upset her tidy mind. With barely perceptible motions, she beckoned me to close the book and put it away inside my handbag. A mere two gestures and her sign language had come to an end: this was the last movement of her hands anyone saw.

During the first night at the hospital I had taken some photographs of her while she slept. The next day, when she smiled at me, I asked if she'd mind my taking a picture of her face. I knew she hated Hetty or me taking pictures of her when she was looking disheveled.

"All right," she whispered as she smiled at the camera, but her eyes were even then death-haunted. Now I took pictures of her hands, resting elegantly on the sheets as the fan made a soothing whirring above. Then I went back for a short nap and she relapsed into silence.

I dozed off into a bizarre dream. I seemed to slide into a sky of incredible pinks, oranges, and purples. I felt my body drifting in midair on a wisp of cloud, floating through timeless space among colors I could almost touch, the same colors I had seen in the sky that first day I was called to the hospital. It was silent and peaceful yet intense; the colors became more and more vivid, inviting me to go on with my voyage. I had the feeling of being higher than I had ever been, and for a few brief moments I had the sensation of dying and entering heaven.

I woke at the sound of footsteps. Harold had come to say farewell to his aunt before catching the seven o'clock train back to Germany. The two of them looked at each other for a long time. Her eyes took in everything, but her words no longer came. Two nurses came to give her morphine: they noted that her breathing had become quite irregular, checked her faint pulse, took her blood pressure.

Hetty returned, with a basket full of goodies for which my mother would have no use. The poor woman was distraught; her companion was about to leave this earth. My own Dia was on her way—I had called and asked her to hurry as I watched my mother's body start to twitch: first her shoulders, then her legs. The odor of death was all around us.

Shortly after Harold left, my mom began to breathe harder, as if it were she who had to catch the last train. She lay on her back against the big, white pillows, gazing at the ceiling, neat and tidy (the nurses had washed her a few hours earlier). It was frightening to hear the pumping of her lungs, and I feared that her poor little heart could not take it any longer. Yet there was still strength in her worn-out body.

Dia had quietly walked into the room and sat at the foot of the bed, while Hetty and I sat on each side holding Mother's hands ever so gently. I gestured Dia to call the nurses, as this beginning of my mother's journey was likely to take some time and I did not dare to leave the room. An older, more senior nurse tiptoed in to join her pretty young colleague, who had clearly never before witnessed a death. She looked like a younger version of myself. *"Vrouwtje, kalm aan maar,"* she told my mother softly, again and again: *Sweet woman, do take it easy.*

The older nurse declared that this was one of the most beautiful departures of a family member she had ever seen, so peaceful and in perfect harmony with all of us around her. So often people died in a coma, or in agony, their relatives bickering over inheritances, forgetting that the dying person could hear everything until the very last moment.

The younger nurse took my mother's wrist but found no pulse. Yet still she was gasping and heaving, as though even now she could hold on to life. Then, incredibly, she opened her eyes wide, with the most beatific expression on her face I had ever seen. The last rays of sunshine through the half-opened curtains shone into her eyes, and for the first time I saw the lenses she had had inserted after the removal of her cataracts, their color changing from blue through gray and green to a shade of purple. As her pupils dilated like a cat's, I knew she was following my own dream road, seeing the same colors. She seemed wholly at ease, relaxed and glad to be on her journey at last. But her breathing was so heavy that I put my hand on her chest and begged her to no avail, to slow down. The tranquillity of her features during that fierce struggle, the disappearing of every wrinkle, and those amazing changing colors were unforgettable. As her skin turned white, a nurse told me to check her legs and hands, and indeed there were white and light blue spots as death crept upon her.

I suddenly remembered the words of a good friend. "At the moment your mom is about to leave you, please let her go, and tell her how much you love her too." I leaned forward, gazing in fascination into my mother's eyes and said:

"Mommy, please take it easy. Slow down, let go. You may go now. We all love you. We are all with you."

Perhaps she heard me, for her eyes blinked, and her breathing slowed to normal. Then it became slower and slower, and a tear rolled down from a corner of her eye. The nurse whispered softly that the moment was almost here. Her body became less agitated, and a faint smile appeared on her face as she breathed her last. It was quarter past seven, exactly one hour after she started her final journey, still with that blissful expression.

The nurses shook our hands and expressed their condolences, then left to summon the doctor to formally confirm the cause of death. I picked up my camera and took half a dozen pictures of my mom with Hetty, and Hetty took some of me, lovingly holding my mom's face. I wanted to preserve forever that radiant expression even in death. Only now did I understand the word *heavenly*.

I came into this world on June 15, 1943, at 7:15 A.M. My mother left it at 7:15 P.M. on July 8, 1999, Hetty's seventy-third birthday. It was one she will never forget.

We cried through the fifteen minutes we were left alone with her body. Then the nurses returned, the younger with tears in her eyes. The moment came to say farewell, but after Dia and Hetty left the room I insisted on staying to watch the nurses wash and clean her body before it was sent to the mortuary. Fascinated as I have always been by death, there was no part of it I wanted to miss.

Her body, naked now, lay before me as I stood behind the bed to take in all that was going to happen. I watched those eyes, restored to teenage blue, being closed. Wearing white rubber gloves the two nurses brought a bucket full of wet washcloths and set about washing her back, her arms and face, even cleaning out her mouth with a special brush. I asked them to insert her upper dentures, but her mouth had already started to stiffen and the two of them were barely able to open it wide enough to insert the dentures.

My mother's body was tossed from left to right, her limbs hanging limp over one side of the bed, then the other, her eyes half opening, her mouth slightly agape. She had become a rubber doll, bereft of the dignity she had cherished so throughout her life. After the nurses succeeded in inserting her dentures, they finally closed her eyes and mouth. When I lent a hand to help them, I felt how cold her skin had turned; the flesh on her belly felt like parchment. Then came a most challenging moment: I watched the nurses wash my mother's vagina. I was amazed at how young and beautiful it appeared. And since after all it had been where I had come from, I thought, why shouldn't I take a good look at it? I even recognized a similarity between hers and my own.

At last, after using pieces of cotton wool to prevent any fluid leakage from the body, they slipped on a pair of underpants, and I helped finish dressing her. She looked once more at ease in the jacket I had chosen for her, and I picked out a silk blouse and matching scarf for her to wear at the viewing.

BACK HOME, our great friends welcomed us with open arms, warm hugs, and tears; the excited animals licked my cheeks dry. Christopher had lit a dozen candles, filled the air with the solemn music of Pachelbel, and placed a few large portraits of my mom and me on the table among lovely flowers. I was truly warmed to have such consoling friends and housemates waiting for us.

Christopher had helped me finish the booklet I planned to send along with the cards announcing her death. Now I was amazed at how deeply he had become involved in our sorrow. I cried against his small-framed body—he reaches only to my shoulders—and then lay down on the couch in the living room. For the next half hour I simply could not stop the flow of tears.

PART I

I

The Medic and the Model

OF COURSE I was not present at Tanya's party; it happened
before I was born. Yet my mother, Germaine, described it to me
often, and so vividly that I can visualize everything that happened
as if it were taking place before my eyes.

Tanya was an elegant woman of Russian and Indonesian stock,
with all the vivacity of the former ballerina she was. She was married to Boelie, a doctor who practiced in Holland and Indonesia,
and they maintained luxurious houses in Amsterdam and the
Indonesian city of Surabaya.

War clouds were looming in Europe, but a wealthy couple in
Amsterdam could live in some style and turn a blind eye to the
tragedy in which they would so soon be engulfed. They loved giving parties, but this one would be special. The guest of honor was
one of Boelie's medical colleagues, a close friend on sabbatical from
the hospital he headed in Surabaya.

"You must come and meet Mick," Tanya told Germaine. "He is
a fascinating man, a psychiatrist and an author. He is on his way to

Paris to work on a novel. Your mother is French, isn't she? Isn't Paris where you grew up?"

The two women had become friends after Tanya, who delighted in expensive clothes, had attended a fashion show in the prestigious Hirsch department store in the Leidseplein. Germaine had been the star model, modeling the winter collection of the designer Max Heymans.

"Yes," Germaine replied with a rueful smile. "But we lived in Germany. And you know better than anyone what they did to me."

Germaine had spent the first five years of her life in Paris—home of her mother, Christine—and still possessed a French passport. But the family had moved to Cologne, where her father, a Prussian, became a well-known furniture maker. Matthias Schluetter was a proud, dominating man, but he spoiled his only daughter—his little Meni, as he used to call her.

Eventually, though, Matthias found himself powerless to protect his daughter when she committed the ultimate sin in Hitler's Third Reich. Germaine started to go out with a friend of her father's named Yigal: a Russian Jew. Although he was quite a bit older than she, eventually the couple decided to marry. As a nonperson, Yigal had already had his passport confiscated. With the threat of violence all around them, Germaine panicked and ran out of the wedding. But it was too late: a gang of brash, brown-shirted teenage bullies cornered her. My mother was stoned and beaten; her head was shaved; and she was forced to parade wearing a notice bearing the words JEW WHORE.

Shocked and humiliated, her family smuggled her out to Holland to stay with her mother's sister in Nijmegen and recover. A fashion designer with her own business, her aunt introduced my mother to a busy and ambitious photographer. Soon Germaine, a strikingly beautiful young woman, had an impressive portfolio and decided to move to Amsterdam to pursue her modeling career. She rented a small apartment. Then she met Tanya, who wanted her to move into the palatial mansion where she and Boelie held court. But Germaine refused; her newly won freedom was too dear to her.

"SO YOU WILL come tonight," Tanya cajoled. "I want to show you off."

Intrigued by Tanya's enthusiasm over this mystery guest from the exotic Orient, Germaine agreed. Indonesia might be a second home to her Dutch friends, but to her it was as remote as the Wild West or the mountains of the moon.

At about the same time, Boelie was having a drink with Mick, the man in question. "All our old pals should be coming tonight, but there is somebody new, a friend of Tanya's, whom I think you will really appreciate."

Mick smiled. "You mean yet another pretty girl?"

"She's something special. Got a touch of Garbo about her."

"Sounds interesting," Mick said.

"Yes, well, she is one of the most sought-after models in the country. Come to think of it, she looks more like Marlene Dietrich. Has that cool, sophisticated look. You like blondes, don't you?"

"This I must see," Mick said. "Perhaps it is time for a change."

Boelie's reference to blondes was sly: he knew that back in Surabaya this highly eligible doctor was surrounded by a legion of dark-skinned, black-haired young women eager to entrap him by seduction or sorcery. He also knew that Mick had been married once before, to a blonde who had borne him a daughter. They had been divorced for more than a year.

That evening, Tanya's salon positively glittered. Old friends greeted one another amid a constant flow of good conversation and good wine. Tanya's taste was exquisite; it showed in the flowers, the food, and that buzz of excitement that marks a successful party. Germaine was the center of attention. She wore a long sequined evening gown, cut very low over her bust. Her perfume, Mitsouko, was alluring yet not overpowering, and her long white gloves were never once removed throughout the evening.

And ever at her side was Mick. Suntanned, with a thick mop of black hair combed back in the Rudolph Valentino style and a neatly trimmed mustache, he wore an immaculate white tropical suit with a colorful foulard wrapped nonchalantly around his neck. She found him to be a lively companion, ready with a joke or some shrewd comment, and their laughter filled the room. Wherever she went he followed, and his dark piercing eyes never left her for a moment. In her presence all the Dutch women he knew seemed dull, almost lifeless. He was determined to possess this fascinating creature, and she was as attracted to him as a moth is to a flame.

What was there about this man that made him so different from all the Dutch men she knew? It wasn't just the trace of Indonesian blood in his veins; plenty of the men in the room had that. Tanya had remarked that Mick was Jewish. *Why am I such an idiot?* Germaine scolded herself. *I run away from one Jew because it meant so much trouble, only to fall in love with another.*

"And what is so special about me that attracts them, attraction of opposites, blonde women and black-haired men?" she asked Tanya.

"No, darling. You are the forbidden fruit, the *shiksa* whom the good Jewish boy dares not bring home to Mama. You are the dream mistress of the husband condemned by the family—especially by Mama—to marry the good, down-to-earth, virtuous Jewish wife who will make him a nice, comfortable home and raise the kids."

By two o'clock Germaine knew it was time to leave, but she found it difficult to make it through the door. Not that she felt drunk, although her glass had mysteriously refilled whenever she emptied it. Perhaps that explained the odd sensation she felt: even as she was standing absolutely still the room insisted on slowly rotating, so the door was never where it ought to have been. Displaying his medical skills, Mick gently held her arm and walked her round the room until it reverted to its usual motionless state.

He prescribed a cup of strong coffee, and he informed his patient that he could not permit her to go home alone. Brushing aside her feeble protests, he ordered a taxi. Germaine kissed Tanya and Boelie good night and thanked them for a wonderful evening. There was a hug and a kiss for Mick, with a wink and a knowing smile. When Tanya wished him good luck, Germaine wondered what she meant; taking a cab in Amsterdam hardly qualified as a hunting expedition. Or did it? She was conscious of the envious eyes of the other women glaring at her as the dashing doctor took her arm and guided her to the waiting taxi. The party was over, but the evening was not.

IN THE TAXI, Germaine said that she felt better; all she'd needed was a little fresh air. But now the motion of the vehicle caused her head to rest against her escort's shoulder, and somehow each time she straightened up it came to rest again. But Mick did not seem to object.

Then, without any warning, he took her gloved hand in one of his; with the other he cupped her chin, looked into her eyes, and spoke to her in perfect German. *"Germaine, du wirst meine Frau":* Germaine, you will be my wife. Germaine recoiled in horror. It wasn't so much the prospect she objected to but the effrontery of this complete stranger who had dared to use the familiar *du* instead of the formal *sie*. In icy tones she informed him that, since they had not been at school together, he should remember that a gentleman owes a lady more respect.

Mick took the rebuke as if she had slapped his face. Her scorned suitor withdrew into the corner of his seat, and uttered not another word until they drew up outside Germaine's apartment. Instructing the driver to wait while he saw the lady to the front door, he helped her down from the taxi. At the door he bade her farewell, drew her glove to his lips, and kissed the middle finger. Thinking that perhaps she had been too severe with this man who

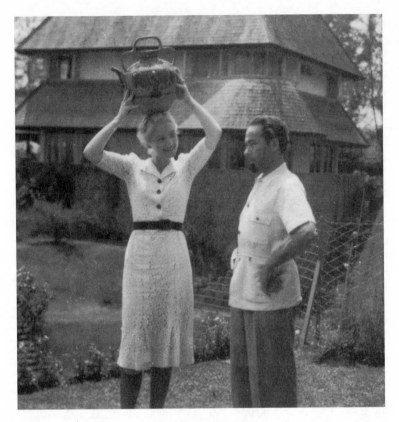

My parents in 1943

had looked after her every need all evening, she took off her glove
to allow him the privilege of kissing her naked hand. At that, the
couple embraced long and passionately, as the meter ran in the taxi.
Germaine never told me that he gave a slight bow and clicked his
heels as he left, but I have always imagined him doing so.

A month later they were honeymooning in St. Moritz.

A WHIRLWIND COURTSHIP leaves little time for an elaborate
wedding; luckily, Tanya and Boelie were on hand to act as witnesses.

Nearly all of Mick's family were in Indonesia, and his introduction
to his future in-laws had been by telephone, but Matthias and
Christine came from Cologne to support their daughter and get a
view of her debonair husband. Matthias was well pleased and
beamed with pride, but his wife was troubled at the prospect of a
long separation from their daughter once she was whisked away to
remote Indonesia.

I was a teenager when I heard some of these stories, so of course
I wanted to hear all about the consummation of their marriage, but
Germaine was far too modest to discuss such matters with her
teenage daughter. She became a great deal more open-minded and
tolerant after she read *The Happy Hooker*, but by then she was far
more worldly than the wide-eyed young bride for whom an entire
new world was about to be revealed by her sophisticated husband.
He was fifteen years her senior—years during which he'd enjoyed
a bohemian lifestyle to which Germaine was soon to be initiated.

"The hotel was very luxurious," she reminisced. "I had never
been inside such a place before."

"What about the bedroom?" I asked in my most innocent voice.

She knew me too well to fall for such false naïveté. "And the
restaurant—oh, it was so romantic! Candles on each table. Gazing
through the window, I had my very first glimpse of the Alps—so
majestic, towering above the little town!"

Perhaps all children are mystified trying to visualize how their
parents made love, and made them. I couldn't have cared less about
the splendors of the Swiss landscape; I was aching to hear about the
intimacies of those first nights together.

But my mother was in a sentimental mood. "I loved those
mountains once we got out on the ski slopes," she said. "And your
father bought me wonderful outfits. You would have loved those
clothes, Xaviera. Everyone looked at me—I felt so proud. And
soon I became a really expert skier. That was one thing I did much
better than Mick—he never had my physical agility."

"Not even in bed?" I ventured.

My mother frowned. "I am talking about skiing," she reminded me. "I had my own private instructor. He said I was his star pupil. He was very handsome, quite dashing, and he flirted with me out-rageously."

I gave her an inquiring look and she giggled, as though she were still the sparkling young woman.

"Tell me more," I urged. Maybe those mountains were interest-ing after all.

"There's nothing to tell," she said. "He wanted to date me, but I was never unfaithful to your father. But when Pappi wasn't around, he took a lot of trouble correcting the way I stood or held my poles. You know, he used his hands rather a lot."

"You mean he would fondle you?"

"No, we never went that far. It was quite innocent, really. I just felt . . ." She hesitated, as if searching for the right word.

"What?"

"I don't know. Perhaps I did encourage him, though of course I never intended for anything to happen."

"Wasn't Pappi jealous?"

"No, no, no!" Germaine protested indignantly. "Why should he be? There was nothing to be jealous about. Anyway, I was very dis-creet. I'm sure he never knew. Although he did make a few com-ments about the masseur."

"Masseur? You mean you were carrying on with *another* man, besides the ski instructor?"

"He was an Austrian, blond and very good-looking." There was a fond smile on her lips as she relived the past. Then she remem-bered herself.

"Don't be ridiculous, Xaviera, I never carried on with any man after we were married. But I was a pretty young bride; it was quite normal for men to take notice of me. And Pappi was very proud of me: he liked to show me off, holding my arm as we swept into a chic restaurant, or just parading down a main street. While we were there, he bought me two magnificent diamond rings. You know how slender my fingers are, and those rings really sparkled in that dazzling sunlight. And if he had been jealous of the ski instructor, do you think he would have bought me such glamorous ski suits?"

Remembering that conversation many years later, I found that touch of harmless vanity appealing: it helped me remember my mother not as an old woman enfeebled by sickness but as a lovely girl, barely out of adolescence, glowing with health and gazing in wonder at the world she was discovering. Despite her flirtatiousness, Germaine was rather naive. The only thing she consented to tell me about her wedding night was what she called the "trouble with the shoes."

"But Pappi bought you all kinds of jewelry and expensive clothes. You don't mean to say he wouldn't buy you smart shoes? Or were they just uncomfortable?"

"No, it was nothing like that, Xaviera. You know what a generous man your father was, but I was too embarrassed to let him come with me when I went shopping for shoes."

I tried to visualize my father making a big deal over anything in a shoe shop but failed. What could my mother be getting at?

"He wasn't a foot fetishist," I ventured.

Germaine was outraged. "Certainly not. How could you even think such a thing? No, you must remember what small feet he had, very dainty, unusually delicate for a man. I didn't want him to notice that my feet were so much bigger than his. Now, I had never stayed before in a hotel where you left your shoes outside the room and they would be cleaned for you. So on that first night I thought it strange that Daddy opened the door and placed our shoes outside. When I was sure he was sound asleep, I tiptoed to the door and peeped outside. There were our shoes, side by side, and I was horrified at how much bigger mine were."

"No, Mamma," I protested. "Your feet aren't that large, are they?"

"Well, they're size ten." She smiled wryly. "Your dad's were eight. I thought, maybe if I don't put them quite so close together, he won't notice the difference, so I moved them apart, to opposite sides of the door."

"So what did Daddy say in the morning?"

My mom shrugged her shoulders. "We decided to have breakfast in our suite, so Pappi called room service. There was a knock on the door, and while Pappi brought it in I straightened up the table. But as soon as he opened the door, he called out: 'Germaine, what on earth have you done with our shoes?'

" 'What's the matter?'

" 'I left our shoes here together to be cleaned. Now I see you've moved yours to one side. Why would you do that—didn't you want them cleaned?' "

Flustered at being caught, my mom tried to bluster her way out of the situation.

"They're my shoes—I can do what I like with them."

"Listen, my darling, we've just gotten married. Why? Because we want to be together, and we want everybody to see that we're together. Shouldn't our shoes be together too? It's a symbol of our very unity that our shoes be together!"

"You know, Xaviera," she told me with a sad smile, "little things like that can lead to dreadful rows, all over nothing. But your father was such a wise man. He just kissed me."

"And you?"

"I was so relieved. That was when I realized he couldn't possibly mind that my feet were bigger than his. Still, though, I was always happier going into shoe shops on my own."

2

Mick Remembered

IN THE 1970s I went back to the house where I was born. We had left Indonesia when I was almost three years old, so I had no conscious memory of my first home. I was curious to rediscover not only my own roots, but—even more intriguing—those of the young Mick and Germaine, who had arrived in Surabaya thirty-one years earlier. My father had been dead for some time, yet I still missed the warmth of his presence, and I never ceased yearning to find a reincarnation of his character in the men I met. He had been so magnificent, so multitalented; in my eyes he was a heroic figure, his life an epic, and his lingering illness and death felt like a crime. So it was natural that I should want to reach back and cast light on those years of his life, hidden beyond the reaches of my memory.

Memory can play strange tricks. As the taxi drove along the street (which had been transformed since the days when we lived there), I envisioned a dream house, just what I imagined our home to have been. Then, suddenly, I recognized it, modest yet stately, standing in a lush, well-tended garden. The driver was looking out for house numbers, but I called out to him to stop. It simply *had* to be that house—and it was.

As I walked up the path a whole pack of dogs started to bark furiously, as if to deny me access to my past. Fortunately, the statuesque woman who opened the door could not have been more welcoming.

"My name is Vera de Vries," I said. "I am the daughter of Dr. Mick de Vries, who used to live here before the war."

She put her hand to her head. Then her face lit up with a smile, and she exclaimed in surprise, *"Adoe!"* Her voice was rich and melodious. "So you are little Vera! You won't remember me; how could you, you were far too young when you all went back to Holland. But I remember you and your parents. Tell me, how is Mick?"

I noted that she hadn't asked after Germaine, and the thought flashed through my mind: was there a hint of female jealousy? She was still quite a good-looking woman, her thick white hair pinned up with an enormous golden hairpin and two elegant ivory sticks, her face smooth and unwrinkled. Thirty-odd years ago she might have been strikingly sexy, with the flawless dusky skin and big soulful eyes of a young Indonesian beauty. When I told her Mick was dead, she was quite distressed.

"I am so sorry, he was such a lovely man," she said. "Now that I look at you more carefully, I can see that you have his eyes." But I could sense that it was the man in the past, not the woman in the present, she was seeing before her.

She guessed my thoughts. "We all loved Mick. He was so alive and witty. There's no harm in telling after all these years: my sister was madly in love with him. In fact, there was an affair—it lasted quite a while, several months. But of course that was before he married. Once Germaine arrived, there was nothing like that anymore."

I wondered. Her reassurance seemed too much like an afterthought. And now I began to remember things Germaine had told me, or perhaps things I had overheard as a child without really understanding.

After their honeymoon, Mick would return to this house and to his work in the hospital across the road. And Germaine? Odd scraps of overheard conversation, unfinished whispered sentences, and one shared confidence of my mother echoed in my mind.

GERMAINE'S MOTHER, Christine, was a happy, good-natured woman, despite years of suffering from injuries she sustained after falling off a commode when a baby. This day, however, Christine *la commandeuse*, as her family jokingly dubbed her, was distinctly unhappy. She turned to her husband and gestured at the letter in her hand.

"It's from Meni," she said.

Matthias looked up from the newspaper he had been reading. "Is she still in Holland? I thought she and that husband of hers had sailed for Java."

"No, there's still more than a week before Mick leaves. She is not sure whether to go along or stay behind."

Matthias snorted. "What nonsense! Hardly back from her honeymoon! Of course she should go with him. They are going to her new home. Whatever can the girl be thinking of?" Matthias Schluetter's Prussian upbringing had been more rigid and conventional than that of his French-born wife.

"She is serious," Christine replied. "She writes that Mick has been cheating on her. You remember that they were living in Paris; apparently Mick has gone on seeing girlfriends he had there before they were married."

"Oh, you mean leaving him *for good,* not just taking a later ship. Well, I think we all knew he was a bit of a flirt. You only had to look at him to see that girls would be swarming round him like wasps round a honey pot. And he never did anything to shoo them away."

"Matthias, we're talking about the happiness of our only daughter. What should I tell her?"

Her husband thought before answering. "Germaine isn't a

child, although she is still a bit green. She knew the sort of man
Mick was before she got married. I know it was all so quick, and
she was swept off her feet, but they had plenty of friends who must
have given her a pretty clear idea, even if they didn't actually warn
her off. That couple, Boelie and Tanya, for instance. She went in
with her eyes open—she can't just walk away now."

"I suppose you're right," Christine agreed. "But I shall tell her
to have it out with Mick before they leave. It won't be that easy to
run away in Indonesia, where she has no family, so she'd better get
things clear with him now. He's a respected doctor, the director of
a great hospital. He must act the loving, faithful husband if he
expects her to be the loving, loyal wife."

"There's another thing," Matthias said grimly. "Who knows
how this war in Europe is going to end? The farther that girl is from
Germany, the better. What do you think the SS or the Gestapo
would do to a German girl who, having been warned off one Jew,
went and married another?"

Christine shuddered. "I'll write at once," she said.

CHRISTINE WASN'T the only one advising Germaine to stand
by her man.

"You knew you weren't the only woman in his life," Tanya
pointed out. "He was married before; there's even a child."

"I'm not making a fuss about his ex, that ballet dancer, or about
little Mona. He told me all about that, how she never got along with
his mother. They're divorced; he doesn't see either of them anymore. Living in England, aren't they?"

"That's right. And I suspect Momma Esther will be just as
beastly to you. They were always against marrying out of the faith,
and German blondes aren't very welcome in these times. So it's his
other women who have got you worried? Well, listen, darling, Mick
has his weaknesses, but he is a good man. He is fifteen years older
than you, and much more a man of the world than anyone you've
met before. He can teach you so much—introduce you to fabulous

people, famous artists and writers, true celebrities; he can give you a wonderful life. Before he went to Paris, where he shared a flat for months with Piet Mondrian, he was at school with Sukarno; they were really close friends. [Sukarno would later become president of Indonesia.] So wait until you see the work he's doing in Indonesia. People there practically worship him."

"Most of them women?" Germaine asked sardonically.

"Yes, Germaine, there are women there who would use every black magic trick in the book to take your place. But Mick had the pick of them all, and he's chosen you. Think about it."

The truth was, Germaine was desperately in love with Mick. Her concern was inspired by jealousy, but more by fear that she might lose him. Encouraged by Tanya's cool judgment and Christine's appeal to her sense of loyalty, she determined to confront her formidable husband. She anticipated a furious scene, angry words, and bitter tears, but it turned out to be a complete anticlimax. Mick admitted everything, regretted and repented, and swore that if Germaine went with him to Surabaya he would never be unfaithful to her again.

Did Mick mean it? Probably, but in his heart of hearts he must have known that this was one promise that he would not keep. Did Germaine believe him? Probably not, but she needed to accept his assurance.

So when Tanya, Boelie, and Mick boarded the ship, Germaine was with them. Watching the coast of Holland fade away as the liner steamed out to sea, she recalled her parents' words.

"Every minute we are getting farther away from the war and Germany," she said to Mick.

"Yes, and nearer to Japan," he replied.

THAT WAS THE CRISIS in their marriage that Germaine had described to me after Mick's death, and which came to mind as I continued listening to that quiet-spoken Indonesian woman who recalled her sister's passion for my father so many years ago.

"And you say there were other women who wanted him as a lover?"

"Oh, yes. He was a fascinating man, a real character. And you must understand, Vera, that in those days there were not many eligible bachelors in these colonial backwoods. So many young Indonesian girls had this ambition to marry a European and be carried off to Holland. Even if they stayed in Surabaya or Bandung, as a white man's wife, they would live in a fine house like this one, with servants to do all the work. The little native girl would be transformed into a grand lady. Well, that was their dream and some of them would get up to every kind of mischief to seduce a highly respected administrator or doctor and entrap him into marriage. If that failed, even being kept as a mistress would be a big jump up the social ladder."

"And my father, he would have been a great prize for these man hunters?"

"Of course." She laughed. "But there were plenty of times when *he* was the hunter. He must have needed a woman pretty badly when he came back here after his divorce. But that was before he met Germaine."

"And afterward?"

But I could get nothing more out of her. A veil of discretion descended; she told me she was not into scandal mongering. If I wanted to know more, I should ask Germaine.

I resolved to have a heart-to-heart with my mom when I got home, but the little I had learned in Surabaya brought to life for me Mick's days in Indonesia before the war. I had always envisioned him as the earnest scholar; after he married Germaine, I knew that he was busy writing a book. In my imagination he was always the man with a book under his arm—if not his own manuscript, a novel by Dostoevsky, or essays by Kafka. And now here was a glimpse of the man, not the doctor—the physical rather than the intellectual animal. So women found him attractive, and he was attracted to women. Perhaps I was beginning to find the roots of my own sexuality.

3

Germaine Persecuted

BACK IN AMSTERDAM, Germaine asked me in what shape I found our old home. I was able to reassure her our house was much as she would remember it, but Mick's once splendid hospital was in a dreadful state of disrepair.

"There was still some of the original X-ray equipment, and I saw a few of the old leather chairs, but they're full of holes now, and very shabby," I told her. "The verandas were filled with crowds of patients, with flies buzzing round their bloodstained bandages, waiting for treatment by the hopelessly inadequate number of doctors and nurses. In fact, the place is scheduled to be torn down in a few months to make way for a huge amusement park—a fairground surrounded by shops and restaurants."

She was as depressed as I was by all this, but when I told her that I'd met some of her former neighbors and friends, and that they'd sent along their greetings, she grew quite sentimental. She recalled how, after they'd set sail for Indonesia after their honeymoon, the tensions of politics and the menace of war spreading

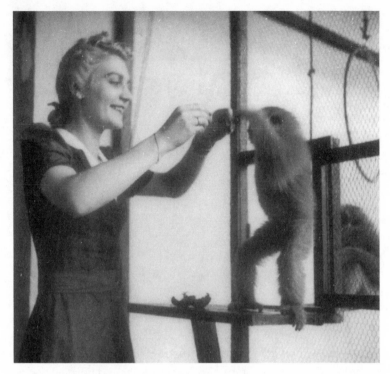

Germaine with her favorite ape, 1941

throughout Europe had seemed to recede. The steady throb of the
engines, unchanging day and night; the immense expanse of empty
ocean; it was all like a warm, snug blanket, soothing and insulating
the voyagers from distant worries. Social life on the ship was a little self-contained world of its own, monopolizing their leisure
hours. Germaine hoped that my father's work on his unfinished
book, and caring for his new wife, would fully occupy his days and
nights. She was disappointed.

Luxury liners have always incubated romances, and perhaps
because this voyage represented a kind of escape from the anxiety
of the Continent, flirtation was in the air. Unlikely couples stole

into each other's cabins, and unattached women struggled to outdo one another in capturing the attention of any attractive man, single or married. Inevitably, a veritable gaggle started fighting over Mick, and he was flattered—and responsive.

"Did he have a real affair—I mean, sleep with any of them?" I asked.

Germaine pondered. "Who knows, after all these years. I don't think so, but he was a damned sight too attentive!"

For a moment she seemed to relive her bitterness, her sense of betrayal, and I shared her anger. She had controlled her resentment, secure in the knowledge that at the end of the journey the passengers would disperse and she would go home hand in hand with her new husband. But new temptations were waiting ashore to replace seaborne fantasies.

GERMAINE FOUND HERSELF the mistress of a whole posse of servants. The role of chatelaine was unfamiliar, but she rose to the challenge. She was the *nonja basar*, the great lady, but her unassuming charm soon won her the affection of all the members of the staff. There was a highly competent cook, much to her relief, and several *djongos*, young boys who did all the odd jobs: shopping, feeding the animals, cleaning the cars, and running errands. But her closest companions were her chauffeur, a serious yet ever cheerful Javanese man in his early thirties, and her *baboo*, or personal maid. From these two she learned of the web of intrigue and superstitious plots of which she was the intended victim.

It was easy for inquisitive women to wander into the hospital with real or imaginary ailments, and keep their ears open for any overheard snatch of conversation. Those who were friends of a receptionist, a nurse, or even a porter questioned them for information about the blond stranger from the other end of the world who had won the heart of the handsome doctor—the object of their own desire. What they could not discover they invented, and her chauffeur routinely brought Germaine reports of the malicious gossip that spread around her.

But what alarmed her most was that some of her most vicious adversaries had found a way of insinuating themselves into the very house, and what they planted there was more sinister than mere words. She first realized how strongly her jealous rivals resented her when, one morning, she found that a couple of glamorous photographs of herself had been turned to face the wall. Their splendid wedding photo had been ripped out of its frame and torn to pieces, the frame thrown on the floor and shattered.

The *baboo* looked grim. "You must take great care," she warned. "They will practice *guna guna* against you."

"What is that?" Germaine asked.

"You do not know *guna guna*?" The maid was incredulous. "The master should have warned you before you came to this country. It is black magic, very powerful. There are witches who can kill with *guna guna*, and these women know where to find them and will pay all the money they have to learn how to cast spells to destroy you."

Germaine wasn't superstitious, but the destruction of the photographs alarmed her. Whoever had managed to slink into the house once might come again and attack the woman instead of her portrait. Later, in her bed, she found a crude doll pierced by pins and needles. She felt sick and burned the evil fetish. The unknown intruder was playing cat and mouse with her. Maybe when she had been relaxing by the pool or playing tennis her enemy had slipped into the bedroom; perhaps she was simply out to lunch, and the servants had been taking their siesta. But what was most worrying was that, although there were several watchdogs trained to attack thieves, not one had barked a warning. Germaine felt totally vulnerable.

And then there was her food. She trusted the cook, but somebody as elusive as her tormentor might contaminate the food before it got to her plate. The maid told her stories of the sorcery native women employed to bewitch some wealthy European—a lawyer or dentist, certainly a doctor—into marriage and sexual submission, slipping herbs and traces of their menstrual blood each day into the man's coffee. She took to eating out in restaurants or her club rather than facing what might be lurking in her meals at home. Such was her paranoia that soon her appetite had waned altogether, and she grew haggard through lack of food.

AFTER FINDING the death doll, Germaine looked carefully before getting into bed at night. Once she found a venomous-looking spider under her pillow; a few nights later, loathsome insects were crawling under the mattress. In a panic, she screamed for Mick.

"What's the matter? You're seeing creepy crawlies, my dear? Typical of delirium tremens," he jibed. "Maybe you should stop drinking."

"How can you say such a thing?" she sobbed. "You know I hardly ever touch alcohol. Look, you can see for yourself. Why do these dreadful women keep trying their voodoo against me?"

"Well, what do you expect when you marry the most eligible bachelor in Surabaya?"

I loved my father, but I have to admit that modesty wasn't his strong suit. Yet if one side of his personality was that of the rational European, the skeptical man of science, Mick's Indonesian roots made him more susceptible to the myths and folk beliefs of the islands than he would readily admit. Perhaps his mocking dismissal of Germaine's fears concealed his own nagging unease. Certainly, his interest in the occult and, in particular, the beliefs and superstitions of the Far East led many of his patients to believe he was a medium, and to ascribe some of his medical successes to miraculous powers.

And it was in the context of his medical practice that Germaine was able to win his respect and that of his patients. For although his specialty was psychiatry, as his reputation grew Mick was increasingly involved in general medicine, even performing operations using hypnosis in preference to conventional general anesthetics. Germaine was his unfailing support, a steadying influence when he was under pressure, the unassuming presence behind the star performer. For Mick was always at work, even when at home. Some patients brought him intractable psychological problems, and Germaine grew concerned at how involved he became in their lives. At meals, even in bed, he was engrossed with finding ways of treating their ailments.

"And that's the way it was while we were still at peace," Germaine said with a sigh.

To hear from my mother's own lips something of how she had suffered in those years before I was born was a revelation, and I felt indignation at the way my father had treated her. But was there another side to the story?

4

Old Flames Keep Smoldering

(Mick's Narrative)

Of course I had mistresses in Indonesia before I met Germaine. There was a sultry enchantment to those sensual dusky bodies. But they were passing fancies. They were all so much alike, not just in their looks—their straight black hair and soulful brown eyes—but also in their mind-set; they might all have been sisters. I had met Indonesian women with brains and personality, but they were older, invariably married, not interested in clandestine affairs behind their husbands' backs—and I could do without that kind of complication in my life too. I was looking for a woman with character, someone with an educated background, with whom I could talk on something like equal terms. That was how I came to marry a beautiful Russian prima ballerina, with a cultural polish with which I was very much in tune.

So I brought this icy blonde into a land of tropical jungles and exotic wildlife—not one of my brightest moments. We had a daughter, which I thought would help bring stability to our relationship, but our marriage was too fragile to survive. To tell the truth, I was still too friendly with

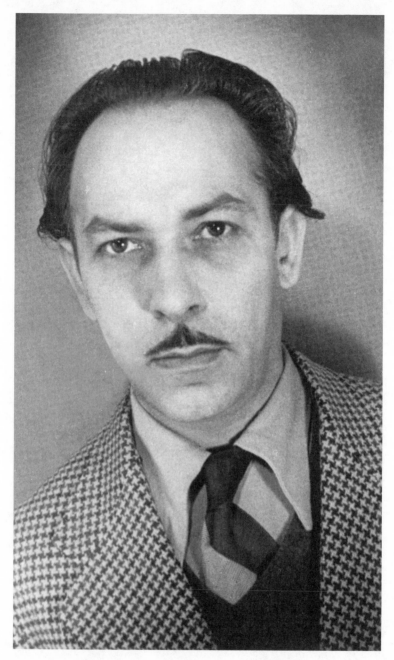

Mick

some women who were only too willing to gossip and destroy our marriage.

But I had reached an age when I wanted to settle down. I had been a ship's doctor, forever on the move; it was a life of fun, punctuated by spontaneous romances that never lasted longer than the voyage. But I had left all that behind when I got the chance to run my own hospital in the city. And then I met Germaine at that party and fell instantly in love. Her female intuition more than made up for her lack of scholarly interests; I could no more lose my temper with her than I could have with a mischievous kitten.

Whenever she did something silly, she was so afraid of my scolding her that she would tell the most outrageous fibs to bluff her way out of her latest embarrassment. Take the way she behaved when we moved into my apartment in Paris, directly after our honeymoon. I call it my apartment, but I shared it with a friend who used it when I was in Indonesia and moved into another pied-à-terre whenever I returned to Europe. As a couple of free-and-easy bachelors we had a great time, hitting the high spots and mixing with some of the great names of cabaret, cinema, and the art world, as well as the garrulous café literati. Not that I went on fooling around after bringing my wife home to the elegance of the Rue de Rivoli. But it was only to be expected that some pretty young soubrettes might drop in casually, obviously hoping for something more intimate than a chat with a respectable married couple.

Germaine found that unsettling, so I began showing off my glamorous wife, taking her out on the town, escorted on my arm, wining and dining her in the most fashionable restaurants and nightspots, But it was quite a culture shock for her to find herself rubbing shoulders with people like Maurice Chevalier and Henry Miller, and she seemed a trifle unhappy at my easy chitchat with Mistinguett—just an old friend, I explained. And of course I flirted with Josephine Baker. She was gorgeous—we *all* were in love with her—and poor Germaine was both dazzled and terribly jealous. But that was Paris. All this gadding about was really for her benefit: it was her first chance to see the world. I'd done it all before; I'd have much preferred a few quiet nights at home to concentrate on the novel I was attempting to write. That was my first moment of doubt about the woman I had wed so precipitously. She was a charming companion, a wonderful wife, a passionate lover. Why, she was even an expert skier. But once I had finally had it with so many nights out, at last I had to put a question to her that nags at every new husband:

"Germaine, tell me, can you cook?"

"Can I cook? Why, Mick darling, I *love* cooking; it's my strong suit."

"Great! So let's have a quiet evening to ourselves tonight and you knock up something simple for dinner, okay?"

Did she look a mite unhappy, just for a fraction of a second? Maybe it was my imagination. "I must go shopping. There's nothing in the house," she explained.

I knew she had plenty of money for housekeeping, so I left her to take it from there. Then, at dinnertime, she emerged triumphantly, bearing the most succulent *noisettes de veau* I had ever experienced, complemented with vegetables cooked to perfection. I was absolutely bowled over. She modestly shrugged off my praise, as if producing this class of food was an everyday occurrence. And so it was. I got on with my work, and Germaine presented me with superb meals, night after night, always a different main course, and invariably cooked with the expertise of a master chef. There was only one thing that puzzled me: there never emanated from the kitchen those delectable odors one associates with the preparation of fine food. But when I asked her about it, she laughed it off.

"Wait until something gets burned or spilled—then you'll have something to complain about."

One night Germaine was about to put out the rubbish, but I stopped her. "That's no work for a woman. I'll do it."

"No, you sit still. It's not heavy; I can manage."

She was staggering under the weight of the sack, so I brushed aside her protests, grabbed the heavy bag, and carried it out into the yard. Among the garbage was a pile of empty cardboard boxes; out of curiosity I turned one over, and read the elegant lettering: Maxim's: The mystery of the odorless cooking was solved, as was the matter of where Germaine had acquired such outstanding culinary skill—her "strong suit."

So by the time we sailed for Indonesia, we were already an odd couple. She suspected me of carrying on in secret with every desirable woman, and I had the uncomfortable knowledge that I could never be absolutely sure she was telling the truth. I caught her out more often than she realized, though always when she was telling little white lies to flatter me or save herself from embarrassment. So there was a tension between us, but it wasn't entirely my fault.

When we arrived in Indonesia, Germaine would amuse herself most days at the country club—which was a meeting place, or rather a watering hole, for a pretty idle lot of layabouts, mostly women who had nothing to do while their husbands were working all hours of the day and night. That certainly was true in my case, and for other overworked doctors, but Germaine always suspected I was carrying on some affair behind her back. To be frank, there were a few escapades she somehow sniffed out, but as I told her, they were no more than banana skins on which I occasionally tripped, nothing to get alarmed about. She was the only woman I truly loved, so I was emotionally absolutely faithful to her. On the other hand, I wondered what mischief she might be getting up to at the country club.

Germaine fell in with a saucily sexy woman called Jane, the wife of a charming Hungarian Jewish colleague of mine, and the two became inseparable, a pair of grass widows. I know for a fact that Jane was stringing along a series of lovers, and Germaine was present at their secret meetings. She told me she only acted as a cover for Jane, but even if that were true, the whole affair was a thoroughly bad influence, encouraging Germaine to have more gin and tonics than were good for her. Worse, taking advantage of her husband's pharmacopoeia, Jane eventually became addicted to morphine. She would become very assertive, totally dominating Germaine and leading her off to all sorts of parties or trips into the mountains with a motley crowd of Hungarians and Dutchmen who had no work to keep them busy.

What Germaine needed was something useful to do, a job that would boost her self-esteem. I didn't yet believe she had the skill or experience to assist me in either the medical or the literary field, and much of the housework was delegated to the domestic servants. The one function that she and she alone could perform was motherhood. And, as it happened, this would be the cause of our most serious quarrel—and another occasion for Germaine to be deceitful, although this time it was definitely for a purpose.

I READ THE NEWSPAPERS and kept up with the international situation, and agonized over the devastation and atrocities in Europe. Like so many other Dutchmen, I had family back there, but I could see that we too would soon be caught up in war. If the Japanese invaded, what sort of a future would await us? Would there even be a future for us? And this was the world into which my dear, loving, foolish wife now proposed that we bring a child. At first I thought she might not have absorbed the ghastly news that was bearing down upon us, so I explained, as though to a child.

I had misjudged her. It was precisely *because* the future was so ominous that she insisted I give her a baby without delay. "It may be our last chance," she argued. "The war might go on for years, and who can tell what state either of us will be in at the end? Give us a child to love and cherish, and give us hope."

I was surprised at the vehemence of her pleading, but not completely convinced. Was this an excuse, a smoke screen, to disguise her true motive? Maybe she thought a child would chain me to her, and prevent my running off with one of those women she found so threatening. She was worried out of her wits by the malevolence of the young native temptresses, who never gave up trying to entice me into a serious affair or even deserting my wife. I assured her that I did nothing to encourage them, but Germaine refused to believe me.

At any rate, there was a bitter row and I refused to give way. I was so much older, more experienced, more in touch with world affairs; surely I was better able to make such a decision. Ironically enough, soon after we were married I had told Germaine that I wanted a child—and she had refused. And not because she wanted to devote her time to her career: in Surabaya in those days, it wouldn't have seemed proper for the wife of a professional man to work, other than to assist him. No, Germaine was enjoying her freedom, the glittering social life around us. Surely she was too young to be condemned to the slavery of motherhood. Now, naturally, I reminded her of how bitterly disappointed her refusal had made me; I've been accused of being a bit of a gadfly, but was that fair? I'd experienced one unhappy marriage, but at least we had a child, and I had been a loving father to my daughter. Yet when I had dearly wanted a son to carry on my name, it was Germaine who had been the flighty partner.

She dismissed the past with a shake of her head. "I'm scared," she admitted. "The war is right here on our doorstep, and I can't face it alone. We might get separated, Mick; I might even lose you, and then what would be left for me of our life and our love? You say you love me; well, then, give me a child."

This was a new Germaine, no longer the pretty little girl I had spoiled, but a grown woman with a heart. But I thought I was the one with the head, so I decided there would be no child until the world had come to its senses and we had come through whatever terrors were in store for us. She fell silent; I took this to be acquiescence, so I suspected nothing when a few days later she suggested we spend a weekend in our country home in the mountains of Trettes. After her nerves were shattered by all that black-magic nonsense, she had been encouraged to take refuge there by that chauffeur of ours. (I say ours, but even though I paid his wages, he and Germaine had become thick as thieves; I'm pretty sure they hatched this latest escapade between them. Certainly Germaine had plotted to get me all to herself, and she and that chauffeur made sure that no one else had any inkling where we were going.)

Trettes was an idyll. We were surrounded by a canopy of tropical forests, the perfume of exotic plants, and the soothing murmur of distant wildlife. The air was cool and so fresh it tingled like champagne, protected as we were from the heat of the jungle by the spectacular cascades of a glorious waterfall. It was a spot designed for seduction, and Germaine knew it. That night we made love, but as never before. She opened her legs so wide, and clasped her arms around me with such fervor, that it was as though she were devouring me. There was no way I could have held back, and she virtually drove me to the overwhelming climax of our mutual orgasm. She seemed to squeeze every last drop of my semen deep into her, and as she came she screamed, "There! Now you've made me the baby I want."

I was shocked, deceived, betrayed. "How could you do that!" I cried. "Are you mad? After all we have discussed, and everything I told you! Don't you understand? Before long—maybe a month, maybe sooner—they'll come for us. We'll be separated, and I won't be there to look after you and our child. How do you think the two of you will even survive?"

But she was unrepentant, even triumphant. She had got what she wanted, and that was all that mattered. "I want your child, no matter whether it's safe or not. I am willing to sacrifice everything to look after it, even if I have to fight to my last breath to protect it. And you know that once you have got over the shock, you will love it as deeply as I do. You wanted a child; now you will have one."

There was no point in arguing. Of course, I was right: the Japanese did come. They confined us in prisons far from each other. There was unbelievable hardship, cruelty we could not have imagined. The strongest of us were scarred for life; the weakest perished. Germaine should never have tricked me into bringing a poor infant into such a world. And yet, looking back after it was all over and sanity had returned, I have to admit that it was she who proved to be right. Xaviera was a few months old when their ordeal began, and Germaine was transformed into a heroic mother. If she had obeyed me, there would never have been a Xaviera. After the war would have been too late—we had gone through too much.

And yes, I did love my daughter—perhaps more than Germaine had expected. But all that was in a different country, in a different life.

5

A Child's View of Hell

FOR MONTHS AFTER the Japanese occupied Indonesia the civilian population remained unharassed, although lives were disrupted and shortages emerged. But fear seemed to impregnate the very air we breathed. Mick went about his medical duties normally for as long as possible, but the stream of sick men and women became a torrent just as the supply of drugs and equipment began to dry up. Despite her lack of training Germaine had become his helpmate in the hospital, one of a dedicated team, but she was gravely deficient in at least one aspect of basic medical knowledge. She had enjoyed a positively radiant pregnancy, suffering not a single bout of nausea, but one day in June 1943 she rose from the lunch table to return to Mick's surgery, complaining of feeling queasy.

"I must have eaten something that disagrees with me," she told Mick.

Her husband hardly needed to examine his patient. "Don't worry about anything you've taken into your body. Let's concentrate on what's about to come out." He smiled at her look of bewilderment. "Darling, you're about to give birth to our child. Come along into the delivery room with you, while I fetch the nurses." And so that evening I entered the world.

Germaine was anxious and fearful after the delivery. She had planned, plotted, and prayed for this day. If her husband were to be swept away in the war's flood of carnage, this child would not only be a living memorial to their love; it would probably also be her greatest achievement. But what if it were born deformed or in some way defective? So before she even asked its sex, her first words were nearly frantic questions: "Is the baby all right? Does it have all its fingers and toes? Are you sure nothing's missing, nothing's out of place?"

"No, no, Mrs. de Vries," said the nurse with a broad smile. "You have a beautiful baby daughter. She's quite perfect, and I'm sure she is very healthy."

Whatever relief Germaine may have felt, though, was quickly subsumed by another reaction, and she looked up at Mick and blurted out an apology. "Oh, Mick, I am so sorry. I know you wanted a son. Will you forgive me?"

But of course she wasn't sorry, and of course he was delighted with his baby girl.

EVEN BEFORE I ARRIVED, my parents had shared their household with a third member: a large, ferocious brown bear Mick kept as a pet. My father was the only person who could approach the beast. He had a special rapport with wild animals—a gift inherited from his father, a dealer who sold animals he caught himself. Knowing the fate that awaited him, on the eve of the Japanese occupation Mick arranged for a local zoo to take the bear and look after it in his absence. Up to that day, man and beast had enjoyed perfect harmony—never a cross word, let alone any violence. Yet now—perhaps out of some sixth sense, some perception of impending disaster—the bear suddenly bit a chunk out of Mick's foot to express its disapproval of its banishment. Mick was reduced to hobbling around painfully for several weeks. But very soon man would follow bear into captivity.

Day after day, Mick went to the hospital and treated the sick. It was he who calmed the nerves of those around him, men and women who had no news of friends or family, swept up in the maelstrom of war in faraway Europe or at their very doorstep. One morning he was examining a patient when the door burst open and a Japanese officer marched in, flanked by two soldiers, rifles with fixed bayonets at the ready.

"Your activities are under investigation. I am taking you to the barracks. You must leave at once. Half an hour to pack your things. Move!"

"Can I have a few minutes to say good-bye to my wife and see my baby daughter?" Mick pleaded.

The officer would not deign to reply, in utter contempt for such unmanly weakness. Yet somehow he was persuaded to grant my father a few moments' leave.

As he thrust a few clothes, a couple of beloved books, and as much medicine and simple medical equipment as he could manage into a bag, my father spoke urgently to Germaine.

"I'm sure they'll come for you and Xaviera soon, so get ready now. Sort out the clothes you will need, collect all the money we have—in every prison there are men to be bribed. Take the diamond rings I bought you, but keep them well hidden. I've heard the women are being confined in separate camps, so God knows when I shall see you again. Be brave, and keep our child safe." He kissed her, picked me up, gave me a hug and a kiss, and told me to be good. Then, with one last look at his home, he hurried out of our lives for more than two years.

For the next two weeks Germaine bustled around, paying off

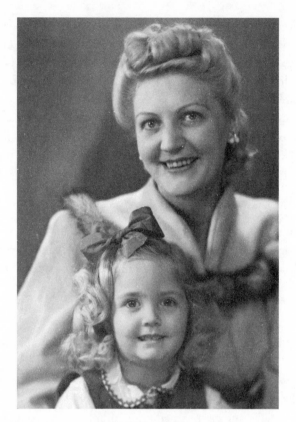

With Germaine

servants, finding homes for the domestic animals—Mick's majestic
Great Dane, her own sweet-tempered silver gibbon, and the lively
little fox terrier that had kept guard over my cot since I was born.
How thankful she was that the bear had already been removed.

MY MOTHER WAS a modest woman. And so it was her more
worldly friend Jane who showed her how to hide the diamonds.
    Jane had been prevailing upon Germaine to accompany her to
those carefree, lazy afternoon sessions at the country club, where

for years European wives had been protected from the harsh realities of native life. Jane was genuinely fond of Germaine, but she was also using my mother, naive and relentlessly faithful as she was, as a cover for her own amorous adventures. Jane's husband had been rounded up at the same time as Mick, along with dozens of doctors and other professional men—all members of the country club. Like Mick, he had warned his wife that it was only a matter of time before they too would be interned. And on that day she happened to be with Germaine when they heard the screech of brakes outside, as a convoy of official cars drew up in front of our house.

"They're here. Grab your things—quick!" Jane ordered Germaine.

Panic-stricken, Germaine seized her diamond rings. "Where can I hide these?" she cried.

"For heaven's sake, woman, where do you think? Up your vagina, of course. They're sure to search you, but with any luck that'll be the last place they look."

At that time there had been plenty of tales of Japanese soldiers robbing and looting, but there had been no reports of women being raped. Maybe they didn't find the pale Dutch women to their taste; more likely, they were too busy occupying Indonesia to bother. Only later would the sadistic fighting troops be replaced by sadistic prison guards, slave masters ready to work their European charges to death.

WITH GERMAINE clutching me tightly, the two women and I were driven to a reception camp. By August 1943 great tracts of Indonesian land had been turned into prison camps, bamboo fencing topped with barbed wire stretched into the distance as far as the eye could see. Though she was frightened, Germaine was glad not to be totally alone, and Jane's wily and resourceful presence at her side was especially reassuring. But the comfort was short-lived. As the women were documented they ceased to be treated as human beings, becoming mere ciphers in their captors' records. After they were allocated to their permanent camps they were forced to march many miles into the wilderness, sometimes trudging hopelessly through savage country, driven off the roads to give way to Japanese military convoys. For the moment it seemed their luck had held; Germaine and Jane were allocated to a building nearby, a former Dutch prison. But it was a big, rambling place with wings well isolated from one another for security, and Germaine was desolated when Jane was ordered to join a group confined to another part of the prison. From that point on the two women would get only the occasional glimpse of each other in the distance. Now it was just the two of us, mother and child.

A group of German liaison officers had recently arrived in Indonesia, and they persuaded the Japanese to segregate the Jewish prisoners from the Dutch "Aryans." Mick, of course, was classified as a Jew, and as his child I was as well; Germaine, untainted by Jewish blood, was entitled to better conditions in the non-Jewish camps, but she refused this "privilege" and insisted on being treated as a Jew like her husband, even though they would remain assigned to different camps. Carrying her baby, she joined a line of women marching into the concentration camp. Over the walls fluttered a banner inscribed with the words BANKSA JEHUDI: Jewish Camp.

The survival of her two-month-old daughter became Germaine's single obsession. With no firm reason to believe she would ever see her husband again, she devoted all her love to me. And yet it was her own body that betrayed her first. My mother had been breast-feeding me from birth and was very proud of the abundant flow of her milk. But now, under the stress of our imprisonment and her anxiety over her husband's fate, the flow suddenly ceased. Her nipples grew sore from the questing mouth of her baby, but no milk came. How could she save me from starving to death? Her periods, too, stopped coming; it was as if her biological life had been frozen, her internal clock wound down. But the only thing that concerned her was nourishing me. Food in the camp was scarce and wretched, but I was too young to take it anyway. In desperation, she went round the camp seeking help. Searching among dozens of women, all herded together, at last she came upon another mother with a newborn child, who agreed to act as wet nurse to me. I would be a teenager before my mother was able to confide in me that the milk of a stranger enabled me to survive. Though the secret had haunted her for years, it did not trouble me at all.

WHEN I WAS old enough to toddle around the camp, I met an older girl named Ankie, and we became inseparable friends. She was a role model for me, a wise old woman at six, and a distant relative to boot: her grandmother was the sister of my Grandma Esther. In stark contrast to my mom, Ankie's mother was a stern character. She loved both Ankie and her younger brother but was ready to give them the occasional slap when they got out of order. Perhaps her strictness explained why Ankie developed a relationship with animals that was far closer and more profound than the normal love of a child for a pet. She seemed to be able to enter into their own world, and when she imitated their calls, I was convinced that she could actually communicate with them.

Unlike our parents, who were restricted to their own prison blocks, we kids were left free to roam all round the camp. From dusk to dawn, Ankie would hang around with the wild dogs and monkeys who had made the camp their home. Like the humans, the animals were starving, and Ankie collected nuts and banana skins to feed them. They in turn grew to trust her and treat her as one of their own. During the day she would take me by the hand and lead me to a lair, where a tribe of monkeys were grooming one another. Since I was with Ankie they took no notice of me and allowed me to watch them, which I did with tireless fascination. The animals tolerated her presence even when they were scavenging and fighting over scraps of food. And together we watched the wild courtships and couplings of the monkeys and dogs.

Ankie was my talisman; not only did she keep me safe from attacks by starving animals, but she also protected me from the brutalities of the guards. The Japanese inflicted every conceivable indignity and suffering on their Dutch captives, releasing years of pent-up resentment against the white European colonists. A number of these savage soldiers loved to fondle Ankie, a blue-eyed, golden-haired child, as if she were their own little angel. Some of them must have been fathers, lonely for the presence of their own faraway daughters; others had pedophiliac longings. But for most I believe she was simply a pet, like a pretty kitten. They would sit her on their laps, stroke her hair, make an endless fuss over her. Perhaps they even believed she enjoyed such unexpected tenderness. In truth, it made her flesh cringe.

Though it would scar her deeply—to this day she has yet to overcome her aversion for all things Asian; she cannot even bring herself to eat Japanese food—at the time Ankie welcomed their attentions, since the soldiers would often give her scraps of food that she would secretly pass on to her starving mother. Her mother prevailed upon Ankie to wheedle a deal with the most amenable of her tormentors—two ripe tomatoes a week for the right to caress. Before long, much to their amusement, Ankie was referring to all Japanese soldiers as "Johnny Tomato."

But the camp commander, a cruel figure named Sonei, was of sterner stuff, not the kind of man with any tenderness to spare for little girls. His brutality was legendary; the word was that he was quite literally a lunatic, for under a full moon his excesses became more frenzied and his sadism descended into rank depravity. Yet one day fragile Ankie confronted this monster, apparently without a trace of fear, and vanquished him.

Ankie's baby brother was sick. The lack of adequate food, and the appalling sanitary conditions, had weakened the resistance of even the adults, and the situation was far more serious for young children. The women had secretly assembled primitive stoves on which they would prepare ghastly concoctions of rice and banana skins; Ankie's mother added snails caught during the night. During one of Sonei's worst periods of cruelty, he learned of Ankie's brother, now a shriveled little boy suffering with the dysentery that was rife throughout the camp, sobbing and screaming astride his chamber pot as his very guts dissolved in an incessant stream of evil liquid. Sonei hated dogs as much as children, and those who lived in the camp had been kicked and beaten by his soldiers until they became as berserk as he was. Now, rather than send the sick child to a doctor, Sonei decided to have him torn to pieces by the maddened dogs.

Sonei's soldiers grabbed the boy and lashed him to his pot. Then he was taken out into the middle of the parade ground so that all could witness the spectacle. The prisoners watched horrified as a dozen or more slavering hounds were let loose to the sound of the soldiers' laughter. Yet all at once they fell silent, awestruck, as little Ankie calmly walked into the ring of dogs, crooning a wordless message to her animal friends. Though the dogs were ravenous, they quickly forgot the target of their aggression and gathered around Ankie, growling softly, some licking her hands before trotting back to their lairs. The soldiers slunk away. Even Sonei must have been shamed; even now I am astonished to realize it, but from that day on he left the children alone and never inflicted any further punishment on them. The little boy survived and became a celebrated brain surgeon in Holland.

After the war I lost contact with Ankie, and my memories of this period were fleeting. Only when we met again decades later, and began to reminisce about those days, did she evoke memories in me that I had otherwise long since lost.

6

Through the Bamboo

IN THOSE DAYS I failed to understand the way women were forced to bow almost double in front of Japanese soldiers, to crouch down bending their knees like frogs. Years later, my mother explained that most Japanese men were shorter than European women; it was an unacceptable affront to their dignity to have to look up to a mere woman, and to stand lower than a *white* woman was doubly insulting. So this posture was a way of abasing the women and emphasizing the superiority of our masters. The women were obliged to accept all kinds of humiliation; the slightest sign of disobedience was punished with mindless severity. A favorite practice was for the man to thrust his fingers into the sides of a woman's mouth and then tear it open from cheek to cheek, leaving a bleeding gash where there had been a mouth. As more and more savage soldiers took over guard duties, there were many who took delight in inflicting torture for its own sake. They would rip open mouths without even the justification of an act of disobedience or a glance of defiance, just as they would inflict beatings as the whim took them. These swaggering soldiers needed their fun, and white women were there to be used and abused.

There was one way of escaping the worst privations, and even getting adequate food: some of the younger women had the option of becoming prostitutes. But I was too young to understand why some women appeared so much healthier and better nourished than such miserable creatures as my own long-suffering mother.

While I was roaming through the camp with Ankie, Germaine struggled to find food for both of us and preserve what vestiges she could of civilized life. Many of the Japanese soldiers relished the opportunity to acquire loot, stealing food or medicine from the camp's supplies to give the women in exchange for whatever jewelry or gold watches they had managed to smuggle in. The soldiers were fascinated by the glitter of gold and silver; it was quite common to see privates flaunting four watches on their forearms. But the main source of the necessities of life lay beyond the wall of bamboo the prisoners themselves had been forced to build, and through which they could never pass.

There were, however, others who were able to pass as they liked: traders. Javanese and Chinese traders were as willing as the Japanese to exploit the misery of mothers desperate for food for their infants, but they generally refused to smuggle anything in: it was too dangerous, and the penalties too horrendous. What they would do, having first extracted whatever money or valuables they could, was throw bags of food over the bamboo fence to the grateful prisoners at prearranged places and times.

Of course, dreadful punishment was meted out to anyone caught in this illicit trade. When one of Germaine's fellow prisoners had a baby who was seriously ill and running a high fever, she pleaded with a native dealer whom she knew to be a smuggler to get some quinine for her. Perhaps he betrayed her to the Japanese; nobody will ever know. But she was caught red-handed. Germaine and the others were forced to watch as the wretched mother was lashed to a stake, doused with gasoline, and set on fire.

Germaine could never forget the screams of that innocent woman, turned into a human torch for the crime of trying to save the life of her baby. But she was soon to suffer her own ordeal.

Something like a year had passed since the dreadful drama of Ankie's brother's dysentery attack; others had since come down with the disease, and not all survived. Then it was my turn, and Germaine was petrified with fear as I rapidly lost weight and tossed in my cot in the grip of fever. She could not get any useful medicine; the best she could hope for was to smuggle in some food to build up my strength. She sought out a Javanese merchant she felt she could trust, and he agreed that, for the trifling consideration of a diamond ring wrapped in paper thrown over the wall at midnight, he would throw back a bag of brown sugar.

Germaine had surreptitiously burrowed a hole in the ground in which she hid those diamonds that she had brought out with Jane's connivance. They would be her last resource to save us in a crisis. Now she crept out at the appointed hour, between the searchlights that pierced the black of the night, and groped her way to the spot in the bamboo. The camp was sealed in silence. Germaine whistled softly, and immediately there came an answering whistle from over the wall. She threw the ring and waited. Then there was a loud thud. The bag had fallen about a meter away from where she was standing and burst open. She could hear the whoosh of the life-giving sugar spilling onto the ground—but so could others.

The camp was suddenly bathed in blinding white light as the searchlights swept back along the fence and spotlights came alive, trained on her as she scuffled furiously to push back into the torn bag as much of the sugar as she could rescue. She heard the pounding of running feet, then the guard shouting at her to stand still or he would fire.

In the prison hut there was a commotion. Ankie's mother peered out of the door, then swiftly closed it. Both her children clung to her in panic. The only sound was the whimpering of the sick child.

"I want my momma," I moaned.

"Shush, lie still," whispered Ankie's mother. "Momma had to go outside. She'll be back soon. Now go to sleep."

They waited. Minutes passed. Then the silence was shattered by the screams of a woman somewhere outside.

"Momma, Momma," wailed the child.

"No, darling, that's not your momma," Ankie's mother said. "Some poor lady in another hut is feeling ill. Now, you rest until your momma gets back."

The screams grew louder, more insistent; the women in the hut shuddered.

"Are they going to set fire to that other lady?" asked Ankie's baby brother.

"Be quiet and go back to sleep," ordered his mother.

They waited. Each minute that passed without their being commanded to parade before another pyre fanned a tiny spark of hope. The screams gave way to incessant sobbing. They waited.

Sonei had been aroused by the hubbub, and Germaine was dragged before him by two Japanese soldiers and one of the Indonesian guards. They did not wait for any order from the camp commander but set about beating the helpless woman. Not content with the agony they inflicted with their clenched fists and karate chops, they lashed her with their belts and batons. Sonei himself smashed his iron fists into her with a madman's fury. She fell senseless at their feet and they kicked her mercilessly, their heavy boots crunching into her ribs and stomach. When her body ceased to move, they trampled on her; one final kick gashed open her face, and each of them spat thick, stinking sputum to mingle with the blood. They left her for dead, sprawled against the bamboo wall.

Early in the morning, a patrol collected corpses and tossed them into a windowless hut with a galvanized roof to await final disposal. They picked up the inert body beside the bamboo, threw it into a cart, and cast it into this House of the Dead. Some hours passed before the flicker of life in Germaine's battered body revived sufficiently for her to open her eyes and slowly become aware of her surroundings: a pile of bodies, some already putrefying. She was dizzy from the overpowering stench of death. Worse, the searing heat of the sun on the metal roof was turning the shed into an oven. Unless she rallied her strength to crawl into the air, she realized, she would suffocate.

Yet Germaine was not physically capable of getting back to her hut and her sick daughter; nor was she permitted to quit the House of the Dead.

Each day more bodies were thrown in, but the guards, finding that she was still barely alive, gave her a little water and some slices of stale bread. But she could not bring herself to eat. She lingered between life and death, growing weaker from starvation and less able to move as her legs swelled from the beriberi that was ravaging the camp. Anxiety over the fate of her daughter cleared Germaine's mind. She knew her own illness was grave enough that without quick medical care she would die—and so might I. When the guards approached with yet another corpse and a hunk of bread for her, she pleaded to be taken to a medical post. They refused. Her voice was no more than a hoarse whisper; why should they bother with a dying woman, already consigned to a charnel house?

But the next day she was still alive, and still begging to be taken to the medical post. After several more days, rather than putting up with her entreaties, they finally consented to move her; she had become tiresome, a nuisance, and they were content to give someone else the responsibility of this living corpse. For two whole weeks, Germaine was in the sick bay. She received minimal treatment, but a little wholesome food; only then was she strong enough to return to her hut to learn whether her child was still alive.

THE PRISONERS who had seen Germaine's body lying by the bamboo wall and then removed in a death cart gave her up as dead; but they had not had the heart to tell her child that she would never see her mother again. Yet little Xaviera incessantly demanded her mother, and each time they told her she must be patient—her momma was coming back soon. What else could they say to a child?

And now I see myself, as I was then, no more than a toddler. I had heard my mother screaming as blow after blow pounded her writhing body. I could not understand what was happening, just that it was something too dreadful to imagine. Then, as minutes turned to hours and then to days, I was seized by the terror of being alone, with no one to provide me with food and above all to love and care for me. Ankie had given me a crust of bread and some water and almost miraculously my fever had abated, but the women were too occupied with their own struggle to survive and protect their own children to succor just one more pitiful orphan. One image survives of me, a lonely, frightened child sitting on a tiny suit-case containing everything I owned, sobbing in terror as a squad of soldiers marched past, each sporting three or four watches stolen from the women, shouting strange words at the top of their voices. *Kirei, kirei:* bow down, bow down!

There was the uncanny sight of a group of women, bowing and frog-squatting, while on the other side of a barbed wire fence, rifles at the ready, these frightening men strode by. I burst into an uncontrollable torrent of tears. Where was my mother? No one came to dry my tears. An orphan has to learn to look after herself. But Ankie went on gathering scraps of food thrown out for the dogs into her apron, shooing off the hungry animals and feeding me the morsels. That was what kept me alive, along with her constant assurances that my mama would be back soon.

So when Germaine at last did walk through the door, I was the only one not astounded by her return from the dead. She kissed and clutched me tight, as if to make sure that I would not be snatched away and that we would never be parted. She never stopped kissing her baby, pouring out her love for the child she had made for Mick. To me it seemed an eternity since she had left, and

I was frightened by the intensity of my mother's emotion. But the ordeal had taken its toll. To this day I remember her strained, haggard look. She had aged years in those few weeks. And Germaine never recovered from the anxiety over her daughter she had suffered during their separation. To literally her dying day she would agonize over whatever I might be doing: whether I was eating wisely, whether I was driving too fast, whether I was spending too lavishly, what sort of friends I had, things that would drive me crazy until I recalled what Germaine had gone through for my sake: all for a bag of sugar.

A CHILD'S CHARACTER is like clay, and my confinement in that hell behind the bamboo wall certainly molded my character. The diabolical cruelty of Sonei, his insane rages, his arrogance—in a word, his inhumanity—are etched with acid in my memory. Yet perhaps most frightening was his irrationality, the unpredictability of his behavior. That Christmas, just one day after he had tortured and mercilessly beaten several women—some from our hut—we were ordered outside. From a radio, there came a stream of glorious violin music.

Sonei told us that we should listen, we could stand straight, he said, or sit and enjoy the wonder of the concert. Sonei himself stood erect. He was an unusually handsome man, and we were amazed to see tears in his eyes as he listened, enraptured. Double rations were handed out to us that day.

The next day we were denied our customary meager rations, and Sonei beat one woman so badly that he broke her ribs.

7

Father Courage

(Mick's Narrative)

When the soldiers came to take me away, I dreaded what would happen to my wife and baby without me there. But soon enough I had my own plight to consider.

All along the road a bamboo fence was being built. Men, stripped to the waist, were weaving the long stems together, constructing an impenetrable wall that would screen the huts and deserted army encampments from the road. All over the island, similar prison camps were being built. I wondered bitterly in which one I would be confined, and whether Germaine and our baby would soon be behind the bamboo.

Of course, as I feared, the Japanese took over my hospital. It was modern and well equipped—not the sort of facility our conquerors were prepared to use for mere civilians, especially detested European civilians. Not that they were much more sympathetic to their fellow Asians, though they did recruit a number of Indonesians to carry out menial duties in the camps, and even to act as security guards. It was clear that they knew all about my practice: I was brought into a building the

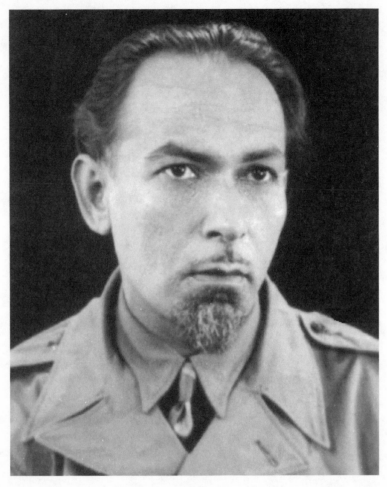

Mick

Japanese had turned into their administrative headquarters, and hauled before an officer, probably a colonel, who told me I would be taken to Ambarawa, about ten kilometers from Bandung, the provincial capital where my elder brother and his family lived. I knew the place was the site of an old army barracks; when I arrived, I discovered that it was now one more prison camp.

The camp commander told me, "You will continue to carry out your medical duties here." Looking through his office window, I saw a group of women digging a ditch. He followed my gaze, and there was the faintest flicker of a smile on his lips.

"Yes, this is a women's camp. But you Dutch don't provide enough women doctors, so we must do what is necessary."

I recalled how many times Germaine had complained about me flirting with nurses and patients. Now I was being forced to live in a whole community of women—but in circumstances neither funny nor erotic.

At first, conditions were better than I had feared. A lot of the Dutch were still free to move around, and although men and women were sent to separate camps, boys under twelve were allowed to stay with their mothers. After a month or so, though, a far stricter regimen was introduced, and nobody was allowed to leave the camps. And we grew hungry. The women were made to work as hard as the men in adjoining camps, starving wretches forced to unload heavy sacks of rice and stagger with them from the railway station to the camp cookhouse. As they stumbled over jagged stones in the blistering midday heat, they were watched every step of the long path by guards, ready to beat senseless anyone rash enough to try to steal a handful of the rice. The grains were unwashed and weevil ridden, but the women were so desperate for food that some of them even resorted to eating their soap ration.

The allotted bar of hard, gritty soap wasn't sufficient for both laundering their clothes and keeping themselves clean. Outside the bamboo fence loitered the Indonesian black marketeers called kedekkers, and the women would sneak up to the fence when the guards were not watching and swap anything they possessed for food, soap, and other basic necessities.

My need was more urgent than soap, or even food. Famine, and the hardships of the camp, drained the resistance of the prisoners, and I was faced each morning with an ever longer line of sick patients. I had grabbed a bag of medical supplies when I was taken away, but they were soon exhausted, and the supply in the camp was woefully inadequate. I appealed to the prison commander and was beaten for my pains. My only hope was not a *kedekker* but a more sophisticated breed of merchant.

Because elderly or infirm prisoners lacked the agility of youngsters, in every camp some enterprising streetwise kids offered to trade through the bamboo for them. This was no act of charity—they demanded two or three times what it cost them to buy from the *kedekker* and grew rich at the expense of their fellow prisoners. Then these *tjatoeters* commenced a secretive trade with some of the more corrupt Japanese, who for a flashy new watch were willing to turn a blind eye to the traffic. So here was a new class of entrepreneurs, dealing indiscriminately with Dutch, Javanese, Chinese, and Japanese. They were criminals, but they were indispensable if we were to survive. I had more opportunity than most to tap into this black market. There was such a shortage of doctors that we spent much time traveling from one camp to another, doing everything we could to ease the suffering of men and women alike. Knowing that I would be transported beyond the bamboo, many of the women pressed into my hand scraps of letters to their loved ones, which I would pass to *tjatoeters* in the hope that some of them might get through. But my main business was to give these shady characters a list of the more easily obtained essentials—bandages, disinfectants, the most basic of medicines.

IT WAS IN A MEN'S CAMP, a depressing array of thatched huts, that I met my supplier and handed him the money I had squirreled away. He passed me a parcel wrapped in grubby brown paper, then immediately faded away. The moment he disappeared, a posse of guards ran out of a hut, seized me, and tore the package out of my hands. I never got a chance to see what it contained.

I knew I was in for a beating and prayed that it would be nothing worse. The commander of this particular camp was notorious for his cruelty, for the delight he took in devising ever more ingenious tortures.

I had been told that men had their stomachs torn open and ravenous rats thrust into the open wound to literally eat the hearts out of their victims. I consoled myself with the hope that as a doctor whose professional skills were needed, I might be spared the worst punishment. Yet my complacency was quickly dispelled when the corporal in charge lashed me across the face with his belt, the buckle splitting my lip and opening an angry welt across my cheek.

My vision blurred as I was hustled into a hut and then stumbled into the presence of an officer. The corporal shouted the details of my offense. There was a moment's silence, then the officer began to question me—and as I gazed at my interrogator I recognized him with dismay as the camp commander himself. He demanded that I reveal the identity of whoever had supplied me with the contents of that parcel. Until that moment, I had assumed that the *tjatoeter* had betrayed me and would be rewarded for his treachery. Now I realized that he genuinely did not know; otherwise the man would have been standing beside me awaiting punishment. On the other hand, if he had been one of their stooges, they wouldn't have been wasting their breath with questions. I said simply that an unknown man had approached me and offered to get whatever I wanted. That was my story, and somehow I stuck to it. Of course I *could* have identified him, and the commander knew it, so he resolved to force the truth out of me.

During the last few days before my capture, as it happened, I had been reading Kafka. Suddenly I was enacting the role of K—but with physical torture replacing his psychological trauma.

I was pushed into an adjoining room that contained a surreal clutter of equipment. One glance confirmed my fears: it was a torture chamber, with the ambience of a medieval dungeon but updated with all the refinements of contemporary sadism. My clothes were ripped off and I was strapped onto a rough wooden bench. One of the men—he may have been a medical orderly—smeared petroleum jelly on my testicles and secured metal electrodes to them with rubber pads. Then the camp commander entered and stood above me. Sneering with contempt at my naked, helpless body, he demanded the name of my supplier. I gritted my teeth and remained silent, but he didn't bother to wait for a reply. The corporal threw a switch, and the pain seared through me from below. My limbs jerked in convulsions, and my bonds bit deep into my flesh. It lasted only a second but then was repeated again, again, and again. I was barely conscious when they tired of their entertainment— but I had managed to defy them with silence.

WHEN THE TRAUMA of short, sharp pangs failed to loosen my tongue, the Japanese released me for a series of new treatments. My genitals throbbed with pain when I was unstrapped; my skin was scorched and discolored. And even the relief of being allowed off the bench was short-lived.

As we passed through the open space behind the prison block, I had a glimpse of other offenders who were undergoing "correction." Two men were hanging from the boughs of trees to which their wrists had been roped, their feet dangling a bare inch or two from the ground. Kafka never dreamed anything so diabolical as this contemporary crucifixion. A few minutes later, though, I found myself almost envying them. I was stretched onto a bamboo frame, to the ends of which my hands and feet were securely fastened. A surly-looking soldier checked my bonds, and then started heaving on a lever, which ratcheted the ends of my dreadful bed farther apart, inch by inch. How incredible that modern, supposedly civilized men should revert to something so primitive as the rack. How many false confessions had been extracted from heretics, witches, conspirators, and simple seekers after truth as their limbs and spirit were broken in the dark days of the Age of Faith and the Inquisition?

Yet this was no time for reflection. I felt each ligament in my body as it was wrenched slowly from my frame. Sweat poured into my eyes, blotting out the hell around me. I heard the camp commander shrieking at me to inform on my supplier. I don't know how I summoned up the inner strength, but I kept my mouth tightly shut, unwilling to give him the satisfaction of hearing me scream or even groan. As the rack turned notch to notch, something inside me seemed to snap. I must have fainted, for I don't remember being released; when consciousness returned I was outside, suspended between the other two hanging men.

Now, though, the brutality of my torturers was working against them. My body had been so savagely broken on the rack that the effect of this new ordeal was blunted. I had been so numbed by my pain that my senses could perceive no additional strain. I guess my tormentors, experts on inflicting misery, realized this, for no one approached me to demand information. I was left to suffer, solely to give them pleasure.

Hours passed, and my body became thoroughly dehydrated in the scorching sun. As evening fell, I was brought down. It must have been six hours since I had been strung up. They had given up trying to make me talk, but before they set me at liberty I was subjected to another barrage of blows and kicks to make sure I had learned my lesson. During all those hours of captivity, however, I had uttered not one word. It was a bitter triumph.

I WAS IN NO CONDITION to find my way back to Ambarawa, so I spent the next couple of days in this men's camp. The conditions were appalling. There were a hundred of us in a long hut, packed so close together that if a man stirred in his sleep, he hit his neighbor. There were insects, even snakes, and our paltry sleeping mats offered little protection. Cockroaches infested the place, but they no longer revolted us. The true pestilence was lice. During the day every man would shake his blanket out in the sunshine and leave it to bake, but at night there would be more lice than ever, crawling out of every crevice. The toilet facilities consisted of an asbestos-lined trench over which we would crouch. Diarrhea was rife, so the stench was nauseating, and some became so sick that they could no longer control their bowels; the floor was at times a river of shit.

In the morning work parties were sent out to chop wood, or work in a nearby paper factory. Others were sent to clean up the huts and other buildings. The worst detail was to dig graves for the four or five men who died every night. I was delivered from this stinking purgatory by the outbreak of fever in Ambarawa, which required every available doctor. Even as I left, I witnessed still more horrors. Passing the prison block, I saw men with their legs trussed up and hot bricks thrust between them, while others were subjected to scalding water being dripped onto a cushion on their heads, forcing them to breathe steam. I wondered whether they would be driven mad by this treatment or, mercifully, die first.

Then: a bone-shattering drive to Ambarawa, a clean shirt, and a line of sick women for whom I had neither drugs nor comfort.

8

Picking Up the Pieces

AS THE WAR came to an end, we women and children were released from our prisons. But such were the desperate and chaotic conditions that the Dutch doctors were retained in one of the camps to offer treatment to a stream of sick and debilitated patients. Among these doctors, still separated from their families, were my father and his friend Boelie, whose part-Indonesian wife, Tanya, had been spared imprisonment. Knowing that they would be parted, and with no idea of what their circumstances would be when they were finally freed, Mick and Germaine had agreed that each should go to Tanya's house to await news of the other and hopefully to meet there.

Until I made the pilgrimage to Surabaya so many years later, all I knew of our life in Indonesia was what I heard from friends of my parents who had shared their imprisonment—that, and the confused and fragmentary half-recollections of a two-year-old. It was not a subject that Mick or Germaine would discuss in front of their young child. But, as I was to discover, subconscious memories of our ordeal haunt me to this day.

One incident does stand out. Germaine, not yet back in our old home and impatient for her husband's return, was staying with me at Tanya's house, whose *baboo* was looking after me while my mother was away on some errand. Even at my tender age I had the beginnings of a tomboy's love of adventure and daring. Out in the garden I deserted my toys—they weren't challenging enough—and set to climbing a gaunt, dead tree nearby. I clambered up onto the stump and managed to climb into the lower branches successfully. But I wanted to go higher, to the very top, and somehow after I reached the next branch I missed my footing. Grabbing at the empty air, I spread my legs wide open, hoping to straddle the branch below. But the old, dead wood was stiff and sharp, and it pierced my skin. There was a stabbing pain in my groin. I screamed in horror at the sight of my blood running down my legs, and that brought the *baboo* rushing out of the house. Seeing me virtually skewered that way threw her into a panic. Seizing me in her arms, she ran to the nearby doctors' camp.

There were two doctors on duty. She began carrying me toward a tall, fair-haired man—Boelie, I learned later. As if driven by some instinct, I struggled in her arms. "I don't want that man. I want the other one," I screamed, pointing at a darker-skinned, smaller doctor with a neat goatee who was standing silently in the corner of the room.

Both men laughed, but the doctor of my choice took me in his arms and laid me on an improvised examination table. At once I felt a strange serenity and the pain vanished. A hypnotic power seemed to radiate from his body; it was as though his dark eyes pierced right into me and into the very wound itself. When he gently opened my legs to inspect the gash, magic seemed to glow from his hands as they brushed my most private region.

"There you are, young lady." He smiled. "It will be a bit sore for

a day or two, but you'll be as right as rain. No more tree climbing
now."

When we got home Germaine was mortified, as though my accident were her fault, though she didn't fail to scold the servant for
losing track of me. Having preserved me for so many months
against every danger, she was terrified that I might yet be snatched
by death at the moment of our deliverance.

About two months after we had been released, my Mom learned
that Mick would finally be coming home. So she put on her best
dress, tied her hair up with a shoelace, and—wearing her only pair
of sneakers—took me to Tanya's house. I can only imagine her
anticipation. When my father arrived at last, I was sitting on a tri-
cycle on the path; his first act was to pick me up and hold me in the
air. "I can't believe my eyes!" he cried. "This is the little blond
angel I operated on. She can't really be our daughter, can she?"
Only then did he run over and embrace his wife. I have sometimes
wondered whether she ever forgave me for stealing her show.

He shook his head in wonder. "Can you be sure it was our child
who came with you into that camp? Our baby had black hair and
blue eyes."

"Don't you recognize your own daughter?" She laughed. "All
newborn babies have blue eyes, Mick. She's our Xaviera—can't you
see how much she looks like you?"

She gazed at me proudly and hugged him with joy.

Tanya's house in Amsterdam, of course, had been the scene of
my parents' first meeting and their whirlwind courtship; what a
coincidence that it was in her Surabaya home they were reunited.
They say that it's a wise child who knows her own father; I don't
know about wisdom, but there was that peculiar attraction at first
sight. And in the years that followed the precocious eroticism his
loving, skillful hands had aroused in me would develop into a powerful emotion, little short of an obsession.

Not long after my father had rediscovered his wife and daughter, the war came to an end. But soon thereafter a new peril arose. Japan's humiliation at the hands of the European colonial powers encouraged the peoples of Asia to strive for independence from French, British, and Dutch rule. In Indonesia things took a violent turn: anti-Dutch rebels and gangs roamed the streets in certain districts, intent on slaughtering Europeans. They signaled by beating spoons against the metal lampposts, and the sound, which became known as *Tingeling*, soon inspired fear among expatriates throughout the region. There was much bloodshed; at the climax of the offensive, there were rivers running red with blood. As soon as we were able, our little family returned to Holland before—like many of our friends—we fell victim to this second war. But no heartwarming welcome awaited us in Europe. Holland had suffered grievously from the war. Life during those early years was grim; having lost his hospital and medical practice in Indonesia, my father had to rebuild his career from scratch. There was some assistance from the government, but it was a meager allowance, and until my father saved enough money to start his own practice again, we three lived a spartan life.

In the months after my mother's death, as I was beginning to write this book, memories of my early childhood seemed to stumble back into my mind almost unbidden. One returned to me when I heard on the radio one of her favorite melodies, the lilting barcarole from Offenbach's *Les Contes d'Hoffmann*. My mother had loved singing the tune in her rich, mellow contralto as we walked through the streets, and one afternoon she was singing that song to herself when a passerby pushed a few coins into her hand. My mom was far too proud to beg, no matter how poor we were, but I had no adult pretensions. A rich aunt of mine in California had sent me a lovely little dress, which I loved to flaunt as I danced about in the busiest places of the city, even in front of the royal palace, in Dam Square. Now I took to joining the organ-grinder who was always in the square, happily tripping to his music; taking us for a joint act, people gave generously to both of us. My mother was embarrassed,

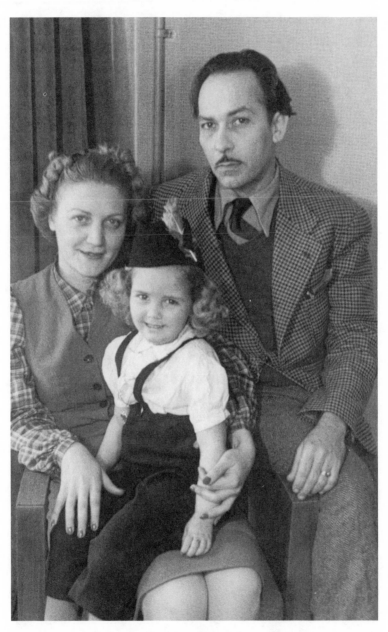

Family portrait: after the war

but she did nothing to discourage my innocent dance-for-a-dime routine. We were hard up, and every little bit helped, so my mother swallowed her pride and accepted the compliments . . . and the spare change.

The organ-grinder was pleased enough to suggest to my mother that I go with him and dance in other spots in the city. But at last this was too much for her to stomach, and besides she thought he was becoming a bit too attached to me, so she stopped our daily visits to Dam Square. My father had just succeeded in launching his new practice, and as he reassumed the role of sole breadwinner, my juvenile act came to an end. And my organ-grinder partner? More than a quarter of a century later he was still churning out his music in Dam Square; whenever I passed, we exchanged a warm greeting.

IT WAS ONLY when Grandfather Schluetter and Christine came to spend Christmas with us that I began to get some notion of how much had been destroyed—not merely in material terms, but in the basic quality of life throughout Europe.

My earliest memory of my grandfather was of his bald head and bushy mustache, curling up at the corners. He had the proud bearing of a veteran of World War I: a shrapnel wound in his leg troubled him so long that in 1947, thirty years after the war, he had his leg amputated above the knee. I would gaze in wonder at his wooden leg, at the crutch leaning against the wall in a corner of the room. In later life, I would indulge a morbid fascination for human deformity, and particularly with amputees—an interest that must have begun with the sight of Grandfather's stump. I clearly remember how puzzled I was when one day he scratched his phantom knee and told me that the itch he felt was a hint that it would snow the next day. He was amused by my bewilderment; but he was a serious-minded man, not often given to idle chatter or romps with his little granddaughter. In fact, I was a little afraid of the steely glint of his eyes, his ramrod back and powerful shoulders. It would be many years before I realized how often those hard eyes had misted over with tears.

He had been a man of some substance, a respected businessman with a solid, comfortable home, when he sent Germaine out of Germany and beyond the reach of the Nazi thugs who had attacked his "Jew-loving" daughter. Now he was practically destitute, a survivor in a bombed-out city, largely dependent on the generosity of my father. In retrospect I recognize that Germaine inherited his determination, even stubbornness, something she maintained almost to the end of her days. It was always Germaine, not Mick, who would tell me off or punish me when I was naughty; it was she whom I considered stern, even tyrannical, and whose attempts at discipline I came to resent. It was undoubtedly her strictness that fostered my daddy's-girl ways.

Grandmother Christine was altogether more approachable, more fun, than her husband. Once their lives had been restored to some semblance of normalcy, we visited them about once a month in Cologne. I remember being fascinated by her immaculately manicured hands, and the glossy nail polish that highlighted the slenderness of her fingers. It was typical of her that she avoided the hard, bright red considered so glamorous at that time, preferring a modest shade of pale pink or even no color at all. And it was Christine, not my parents, who first encouraged me to start thinking of myself as a woman. On my thirteenth birthday she gave me a "roulette bra," a bra with a little padding to flatter my budding bosom. To mark the solemnity of the occasion she donned a new pair of reading glasses; unaccustomed to the sight, I begged her to take them off.

"No, my child, I need them to hear you better," she replied.

That was my grandma, always good for a giggle: in her I found the lighthearted ease I sought in vain in my own mother. Only when my grandma's heart gave out did she confide in me on her deathbed how many times she had fought back her tears in the face of adversity.

As I grew into consciousness, my father became my ideal as a scholar, a philosopher, an author; my grandmother embodied the gentleness and humor of life. But where did that leave my mother? Unconsciously, I shut Germaine out of the emotional side of my life as if she were a stranger, even a rival for the attention of my father. Germaine loved and cared for me, far more than Mick or Christine. It was she who watched over me every minute of every day. Yet her only reward was my hostility. How else could she respond, other than to become ever more concerned with my behavior—or misbehavior?

IN COLOGNE I met the rest of Germaine's family, those who had survived the war—my uncles, aunts, and cousins. Germaine's elder brother, Marcel, had returned from the war in Russia, but he was already stricken with a cancer from which he died three years later. But even as a child he had towered above his diminutive mother. My lasting memory was of his mother forever declaiming, *"Zelli, setz dich damit ich dich einen ums Ohr hauen kann"*—"Zelli, sit down so I can box your ears!" Though everyone recalled her saying this, she never carried out the threat, but the saying became a family tradition. The younger of the brothers, René, was for a time more fortunate, becoming a headwaiter in a very exclusive restaurant in Düsseldorf. But the stress of his work left him vulnerable to tuberculosis, from which he recovered only after six years at a sanatorium in the clear air of the Swiss mountains. His recovery was so complete that he married his nurse, Helma, survived another forty years, and fathered a son, Harold—the same cousin who would join me many years later at Germaine's side during the trauma of her last days. As a child Harold was as horribly spoiled by his parents as I was, and we would compete for who could finish a meal first. It was a habit for which Germaine would scold me until the end.

MICK'S FAMILY also had suffered through the war, but their story was very different. His mother, Grandma Esther, was the matriarch. She had been deserted by her husband, who combined the amiable characters of gambler, smuggler, and womanizer, and had left her penniless with five young children. But the treachery of a mere fly-by-night husband could not destroy a woman who had the granite strength of character to remain uncrushed by the worst brutalities of the Japanese occupation. She was a skillful seamstress and, with some initial financial support from her family, had set up her own business in Java long before the war. So successful was she that before she returned to settle in Holland, she owned a chain of boutiques in Surabaya. She hired dozens of women, Indonesian or more often Chinese, whose nimble fingers would turn out perfect copies of the latest designer outfits from Europe in exchange for a miserable pittance.

Every couple of months Grandma Esther would descend upon our household, to the consternation of Germaine. She was a strong woman with a sharp tongue, incisive and intolerant of anything she perceived as weakness, and on every visit my mother was pitilessly tongue-lashed by her imperious mother-in-law. In my memory she is imposing but elegant, with flashing black eyes and powerful features, forever smoking cigarettes in a long holder. Right until senility struck her at ninety-three she dressed fashionably, with a preference for bright colors to match her scarlet nail polish, and I well remember her eye for handsome young men.

Formidable though she was, Grandmother Esther always found time for little Xaviera. My parents were busy people, and it was Esther who kept me occupied. She taught me embroidery and told me stories, many of them made up on the spur of the moment. It was Esther, not Mick, who taught me traditional Yiddish songs and first made me aware of my Jewish cultural roots.

Still, her visits were fraught with tension, as my poor father struggled to keep the peace between his wife and his mother. To his credit, he always stood up for Germaine to protect her from being bullied, but he must have been relieved when Queen Esther moved on to disturb the domestic tranquillity of another son or daughter. Like their mother, all the rest of her progeny had instantly rejected the blond shiksa Mick had brought into the clan . . . with one exception: his youngest sister, Zettha—Auntie Zettha to me.

Zettha was a short, chubby woman with soft features and a gentle voice; she showed enormous sympathy to my mother, and as a child I loved her, yet she too could be a tyrant in her own fashion. In contrast to her mother's free and easy lifestyle, Zettha maintained an iron-fisted control over her household, strictly enforcing the precepts of conventional morality. She never allowed a dirty word, a sly remark, even the merest innuendo in her house. Her husband, Theo, a stolid, uptight Dutchman who was the director of the important training school for pilots near the Hague, uttered nary a word of protest. But when Auntie Zettha expired at the age of ninety-one, her widower sighed with relief. "At last I can tell a dirty joke!"

And Germaine found another friend in Esther's eldest daughter, Beppy de Vries—the aunt who had sent me my delightful dancing frock from Los Angeles. Beppy was a beautiful woman, sultry in the manner of Eartha Kitt, and with the slinky grace of a great ballerina; she was a talented actress, but her glamorous lifestyle had less to do with her career than with her success in marriage. Beppy's husband, Arthur, was a wealthy diamond dealer in Antwerp before he took the role of adoring husband to this overpowering sex goddess; the pair of them made a deep impression on me whenever they came to Amsterdam, showering us with exotic presents.

Maybe it was because Germaine was such a restrained personality, as opposed to Arthur's outrageously theatrical wife, that Arthur was drawn to my mother; she took great comfort in his understanding and friendship, and grew to see him as something of a champion and a father figure for her—a quality Mick certainly lacked.

I WAS NOT much more than a toddler when we returned to the drabness of postwar Holland, but after the brutalities of the prisoner-of-war camp I was oblivious to the gray hardships of our life.

Mick's splendid career as hospital director was a thing of the past. In place of our luxurious house and grounds, staffed by servants, we had to make do with a dingy walk-up apartment in a busy, unfashionable street. And as I grew up I was initiated into the art of economy by my parents, who kept a firm eye on my pocket money and insisted that if I wanted something special, I should save up until I could afford it. Today, acquaintances are often puzzled by the apparent contradiction in my behavior: I entertain a great deal and spend money freely, not solely for my own enjoyment but also to give pleasure to my many friends; yet in petty matters I will sometimes quibble and haggle over an odd guilder that couldn't possibly make a difference. It is a trait of my character I cannot alter, the indelible impress of the poverty that inhibited my childhood, coupled perhaps with my memories of Auntie Beppy and the gloss and glitter of Hollywood she brought with her. I'm sure I also inherited something of Grandmother Esther's business acumen, and of her dry Jewish humor; from my Auntie Zettha, I like to think, I learned a wonderful sense of fun.

9

Growing Pains

AFTER ALL the terrors and tribulations of the prison camps in Indonesia, it might seem crazy to suggest that my little family had been lucky in any way. Yet if we had remained in Amsterdam, it is almost certain that my father, a Jew well known for his intellectual activities as well as his medical practice, would have been dispatched to a death camp. As he learned how many of his friends and colleagues had died in the gas chambers, his usually ebullient personality began to assume darker tones. The war was a trial from which no one survived unscarred, even the youngest of children. My father might have seen me as a little angel, but soon I began acting more like a little monster. I had witnessed so much mindless cruelty by the Japanese that I had become desensitized to suffering, and I began to inflict horrible torments on innocent animals, pulling the tail of any dog or cat I could find. My behavior is surprising to me even now, especially given Ankie's efforts to teach me to show kindness to all creatures, to talk to them and show them respect and affection. But her influence was not powerful enough to save me from the lingering effects of the sadism that had colored my earliest days.

Brutalizing the neighborhood pets, though, did little to liberate me from that gnawing inner anguish. I lived through suffocating nightmares of marching soldiers and officers screaming and barking commands; always bearing down upon me was roll after roll of barbed wire. My screams awakened my parents in alarm, and my constant bed-wetting continued until I was eleven. My parents tried to save my mattress by fitting a rubber sheet beneath the cotton one, but I became addicted to the comforting wet warmth and even the smell of my own urine, and their attempts to lure me out of my virtual womb were in vain. This traumatized fetus refused to be reborn. To appease my parents I sometimes grabbed the chamber pot and pulled it into my bed; but this only made matters worse, since I would often fall asleep astride the pot eventually falling over and spilling the contents over the sheet.

Even after I was old enough to walk to the toilet, I found fresh excuses for my habit, pleading fear of the long, dark corridor that led to the bathroom. I have long since lost my childhood yen for the aroma of urine, yet as an adult I have often enjoyed golden shower games. And the smell of rubber, so tart and chemical, still brings me pleasure. Any sudden or unexpected noise at night too would throw me into a panic; to this day I need a light in my bedroom until I fall asleep. One of my lovers has joked that the one sure way to wake Xaviera up in the middle of the night is to switch off the light.

As a psychiatrist, my father also recognized the daytime symptoms of my lingering distress. I was forever fiddling about with my hands, unable to find a moment's relaxation. If I wasn't knitting, sewing, embroidering, or writing in my diary, I would doodle—anything to keep me busy. I drove my parents mad, never sitting still, scraping my chair across the floor, whistling tunelessly in the house or in the street. A succession of cleaning ladies complained to my mother about my rudeness and boorish behavior, but she suffered even more than they did.

My parents, it now occurs to me, must have hoped that my rebelliousness would be quelled by discipline once I entered school. But any such hopes were frustrated: instead of pulling the tails of cats or dogs, now I pulled the hair of other little girls. That they would fight back, I found stimulating. I relished the challenge of a fight. I was never a bully, but I became notorious because I was always the winner. The teachers, naturally, found me intolerable; instead of showing me kindness or consideration they merely handed out reprimands and punishments, and that of course only made me more defiant.

There was just one exception: a lovely, gentle, compassionate woman, part Indonesian and a lesbian. Miss May was truly warm and caring, and the sudden blossoming of human tenderness she brought changed my life. I was maddeningly naughty, but I was also the brightest kid in the class, and Miss May had the patience to encourage me. She showed me poems she had written, full of homesickness for the fragrance and colors of her native land, and in later years she gave me records of gamelan music and sentimental folk songs from Java.

Despite the benign influence of Miss May, though, my inner life was a torment I struggled with alone. Without friends at school or in the neighborhood, I longed for companionship from my parents but found it lacking. My father soon was busier than ever with his practice, and my mother spent much of her time acting as his assistant and chauffeur. This one very lonely little girl was left to her own devices in the house, reading books, writing in her diary, nurturing a jealousy that her mother, and not she herself, got to spend the day with her father. During the week, my only time with my parents was at dinner; the rest of the time I spent in my own tiny room, a cell I fantasized into a palace, fretting that I could have been happy with the brother my parents never gave me.

Desperate to conquer my bed-wetting problem, my father eventually resorted to the last recourse of a parent—bribery. He promised me twenty-five cents for each night my bed was dry in the morning. It was a miracle cure; I became a chamber pot capitalist. My father forever after took credit for his psychological gambit, but I wonder whether it wasn't the tenderness and understanding of Miss May, whom I also encountered that year, to which I was responding.

My problems weren't fully resolved, though, until I was fourteen, when I made a series of visits to a child psychiatrist who specialized in children who had survived concentration camps. After he questioned Germaine intensely about the conditions of our incarceration, the doctor put me through a form of rebirthing therapy: only then did I learn to cry, to allow that grief and fear to flow out rather than repressing them within my troubled heart.

MY STATE OF MIND also suffered from tensions between my parents. My father was still the flirtatious Mick of old, and my mother suspected him of having affairs with any and all of his women patients, who solicited his attention at all hours of the day or night. All too often our rare moments together as a family were soured by quarrels, as Germaine accused Mick of spending rather longer than he ought with some lady suffering sudden, mysterious stomachaches and other vague symptoms just when her husband had gone out of town. And that, I realized later, explained why my mother accompanied him wherever she could, hovering close by during even the most confidential consultations.

When I was eleven, my father's infidelity led to one explosion that threatened the very survival of our family. Shortly after Christmas, the old spinster who worked as our bookkeeper asked my mother about the new mink coat she knew my father had bought. Germaine was puzzled: Mick had given her a beautiful fur coat for Christmas, but it was gray seal, not mink. Germaine never used to go through her husband's accounts, but now her suspicions had been aroused. When she looked at the books, she discovered an invoice for *two* fur coats—her gray seal and, indeed, a mink.

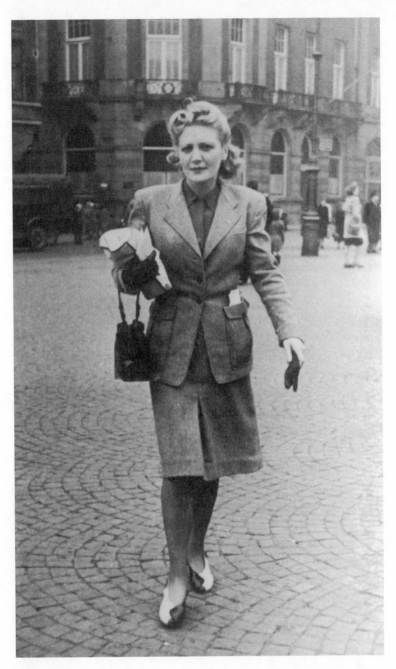

In Amsterdam

Immediately my mother suspected a particular patient of my father's, a woman in her early twenties with a curvaceous body, cheap earrings, and a very sexy laugh. The "mustard maid," as my mother called her—she worked as a packer in a mustard factory—was prone to asthma attacks, usually at night when her husband was out at work. She phoned my father for house calls and dropped in unannounced whenever she pleased.

The scene was set. It was in the middle of the winter, twelve o'clock on a cold, snowy night. I was sleeping soundly when I was rudely awakened by loud noises and screams downstairs. I rushed to the top of the staircase and crouched there, shivering and freezing, in the icy darkness. I peered over the banister and saw the mustard maid running out of the house, her pitch-black hair flopping wildly over the collar of her mink coat, pursued by Germaine's screams.

My mother had spotted the woman, resplendent in a mink coat she could never have afforded, slipping stealthily into Dad's consulting room. My mother waited ten minutes, then without warning walked in. There was Mick, his white coat open; his "patient," naked beneath her fur coat, was bending forward, her head buried in my father's crotch.

"What are you doing with my husband in my house!" she shrieked. "Get the hell out of here, and don't ever let me catch you in this house again, you slut!" She seized the woman, bundled her out of the room, and pushed her into the street, mink coat and all.

Then it was my father's turn.

"That was the last straw," she yelled. "I want you out of my life. I've had it with you. I want a divorce, and *now!*" She marched out of the consulting room with Mick at her heels, buttoning up his pants and trying to regain his composure. I crept down the stairs and peeped through the crack in the door, trembling with fear. I had never seen my mother in such a rage.

My dad was sitting on a horseshoe-shaped couch, before a big round wooden table whose thick glass top was etched with a dozen colorful salamanders and snakes, lit softly from beneath. It was one of our favorite possessions, shipped from our home in Indonesia. He watched as my mother paced furiously up and down the room. Suddenly she stopped and turned toward him, legs apart, hands on her hips.

"*Du Schweinhund,*" she yelled, reverting in her frenzy to her mother tongue. "*Verdammt noch mal, du glaubst du bist ein Üebermensch?* Who do you think you are?"

I had crept into the room, horrified. My father sat silent, as if resigned to his wife's fury. His apparent indifference enraged Germaine even more.

"What is your excuse?" she screamed.

Calmly he took his book from the table and started to read. Germaine went berserk. Picking up a beautiful antique Chinese vase from the middle of the table, she raised it above her head and smashed it into the glass tabletop.

My father's eyes filled with tears, a vision I had never seen before. I was so distressed that I came out of my hiding place, put my arms around his shoulders, and bent over to kiss away his tears. I can still taste the salt on my lips. Mad with rage, Germaine tried to pull me away, but I clung to my father with all my strength.

"Vera, you realize what you are doing, taking his side?" she shouted. "Your father has just done something horrible to me, and I never want to see him again. *Ever.*" She turned on my dad viciously. "Don't you think you ever get to see your child again. She is mine."

"*Look!*"

At last my father had opened his mouth. He pointed at the table. We watched in astonishment as the glass top slowly began to crack with a splintering sound, the engraved animals disintegrating before our eyes, until with one final crash it collapsed and fell to the floor in a thousand pieces.

My father was broken. "I'll *never* be able to replace that glass. Did you have to do that, and destroy our last memories of Java? Did that make you feel good? Are you happy now?"

The three of us huddled round the shattered table and held one another close. We had loved that magical object; now it had gone out of our lives forever. Those salamanders, like the snakes we had encountered on holiday or those decorating his dressing gown, had been as much a part of my father as the entwined serpents of Aesculapius, which symbolized his profession. To the day he died, Mick's favorite ring had borne the image of two snakes, one's eye of ruby, the other's of green jade, biting each other's tails. Years later, flying on mushrooms at the age of thirty-three, I revisited Indonesia to seek out my roots, and the dream of the cracking salamanders returned in a multicolored vision: salamanders, dragons, and snakes danced before my eyes in circles, finally sneaking up my body. In my half-waking state I wanted to stroke the slithery things, but they slipped through my fingers like water or sand until they shattered, turning into a mosaic like the pattern on an Italian floor.

Now, gazing at my embattled parents, I burst into tears, and suddenly they both realized how their spiraling violence was affecting their child.

"Please, Mommy, don't send Pappi away," I pleaded.

She stared at me as if her resolution were faltering.

"Do forgive him!"

She shook her head like someone waking from a nightmare and turned to her husband. "For the child's sake," she murmured. "But never, never again disgrace me like that. Never do your dirty laundry in my house again."

I stood there, hugged and kissed by my mom, who apologized for the way she had wrenched my arm. My father's body was to one side of me, my mother's on the other, and I reveled in the warmth I found between.

Years later I reminded my mother of the scene with the mustard maid. "Tell me," I joked, "why didn't you keep that mink coat instead of sending her out in it?"

"What, send her out naked?" She looked shocked. "I couldn't do that!"

"I certainly could have," I replied.

I'll never forget the expression on my father's face as the tears traced his cheeks; nor will I forget the beauty of my mother's face when flushed with anger.

The following morning my father closed his practice for a couple of days and devoted the time to my mother, cooing and flirting with her outrageously. They made up in exuberant style, taking me out to a lovely Indonesian restaurant, and the three of us went on a shopping spree, spoiling me shamelessly. The house was filled with bunches of roses and boxes of chocolates; my mom was wearing brand-new Chanel No. 5.

Although still a child, I was becoming aware of how close love is to hate, how inextricably linked are jealousy and insecurity, desire and frustration. And my mother's advice I would take to heart: "If you get married, don't have separate twin beds, only one king-size bed. And never go to sleep when you're both angry without making up in some way, even if only by touching each other's toes, or reaching out for each other's hand."

Wise words.

10

Mick the Magician

"A SMALL, wiry man, half-Jewish, half-Indonesian, very intelligent but totally undisciplined and not to be controlled by anyone. A womanizer and an accomplished hypnotist, an excellent actor and musician, highly knowledgeable and much more worldly wise than his fellow students, he was the life and soul of a party." That was my father, in the words of Simon Vestdijk, his closest friend since their days together at college. Vestdijk was mistaken, though, in one respect: although there was undoubtedly Indonesian blood flowing through Mick's veins, and he had absorbed much of the culture of the Orient, both his parents were Jewish. Neither was religiously inclined, but his mother occasionally attended synagogue, and it was from her that he had acquired some knowledge of Yiddish—and, perhaps, his sense of humor.

Vestdijk went on to become the most celebrated Dutch man of letters of his generation, but Mick was in a way the spark that gave rise to his genius. He based the leading characters in his books on careful observations of real people and was fascinated by Mick and his bohemian lifestyle, which so outraged Germaine. His ability to hypnotize animals was the theme of *Dr. Barioni and His Dog* and Vestdijk was so convinced of Mick's powers that he appealed to his friend to captivate pretty young women for his own entertainment—a sort of seduction by proxy!

Vestdijk described Mick's wild mood swings, from utter despair to a manic lust for life, and when I read his words I recognized myself as my father's daughter. As a couple of carefree bachelors in their twenties, they would sometimes settle their hotel bills by paying their hostesses in bed rather than in cash; many a chambermaid was rewarded in a currency older than coinage.

After his marriage, Mick claimed he was a reformed character—but Vestdijk told another story. At the end of their fabulous Parisian honeymoon, catered by Maxim's, Germaine returned to Holland while Mick stayed on for a few more weeks, claiming he needed to conclude some research for a book he was writing. Having observed just how intimate his relations with the female objects of his research could be, his bride had her suspicions, and she decided to confront him with proof of his infidelity and threaten to end their marriage. So she hired a private detective in Amsterdam to spy on Mick and report his lapses to her. Such services don't come cheap, but Mick had generously provided Germaine with a housekeeping allowance, and what could be a more legitimate expense than domestic espionage?

The detective had little difficulty in locating his quarry. As Vestdijk recounted in his diary, it wasn't so much that Mick couldn't resist women, but he was fascinated by whores and loved to frequent the more exotic Parisian bordellos. In one such establishment the man spotted Mick, fully clothed but surrounded by the ladies of the house, delighting them with jokes and repartee. But Mick just as quickly spotted the private dick and came to an amicable arrangement with him: in return for a squeaky-clean report to Germaine, he would be treated to the services of one of the staff and given an additional "financial inducement" to hold his tongue.

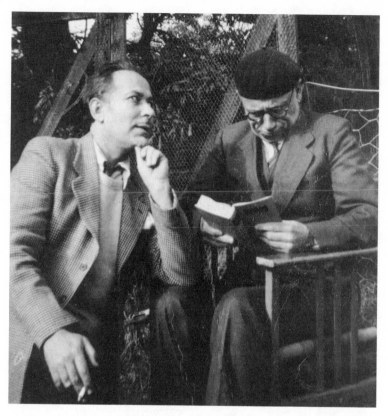

Mick with Simon Vestdijk

In the end, everyone was happy: Germaine got good news, Mick got a reprieve—and the detective, he got paid twice. But there was a more serious side to my father's relationship with Simon Vestdijk. Mick also wrote books, and one in particular—*Arlatine*—was written in fourteen days as a riposte to Vestdijk's adaptation of Mick's real-life sexual adventures in his own books. And while my father was not really a political writer—their shared interests ran to esoteric subjects like alchemy, astrology, and telepathy—it was Mick who was bold enough to confront the legacy of Nazism, with a Hitler satire called *F. Uehrer.* The book was inspired by an incident some six years after the end of the war, when we visited the spa resort of Baden-Baden and stopped for a meal at a fashionable restaurant. My father had let his dark hair grow long, and with his big black hat he looked for all the world like an Orthodox rabbi. When we left, we found our brand-new white Opel Kadett covered with hate graffiti: JEWS HAVE EATEN HERE ONCE—NEVER AGAIN MUST THEY THRUST THEIR SNOUTS IN! JEWS OUT! He ordered my mother and me to get in the car, then began wiping off the filth. Had nothing changed in this country? He vowed never to set foot again in Germany, except to visit family.

BUT MY MOST VIVID MEMORIES of my father's friendship with Simon Vestdijk go back to the times we spent at his country retreat at Doorn. The two men would stroll for hours through the sun-dappled woods, a pair of golden retrievers frolicking at their heels while Vestdijk's common-law wife, Ans Koster, dutifully stayed in their house with Germaine, preparing lunch and chatting. Germaine urged me to stay with them—surely a little girl's place was back there in the kitchen, learning to become a good house-wife, and until I was ten I'd gladly accompanied my mother on all her household rounds. But now, at Doorn, I rejoiced in escaping from the henhouse to join the strutting cocks. I pretended to be too preoccupied with playing catch with the dogs to be taking any notice of my father's conversations with Vestdijk, but as I trotted ahead or dawdled behind them I listened intently as they discussed world affairs and literature, war and recent history. Without fully understanding them, of course, I absorbed their thoughts on clas-sical music and astronomy, was fascinated by Vestdijk's account of his brooding fits of depression and by Mick's psychological exper-tise. Even their casual reminiscences of everyday life in Indonesia captivated me—as did their hushed discussions of Mick's romantic encounters. I heard more, and understood more, of these intima-cies than either man realized.

How fondly I remember that house in the woods. It was a warm and friendly place, as well as a shrine of learning and culture, and Ans looked after it with a mixture of devotion and awe. She was considerably older than Vestdijk—indeed, had been his housekeeper when he was a student—and it wasn't until his thirties that they chanced to meet again. Vestdijk found Ans's kindness and domesticity sympathetic, and her reverence toward him must have flattered his vanity, so after a while she moved in with him.

But the passionate side of his character craved a more exciting companion, somebody on his own intellectual level—and so into the void of his emotional life glided an old friend of Mick's. Henrietta van Eyck was a pretty brunette Vestdijk's own age, light-hearted but a talented author, and her lively and enchanting company was soon complementing Ans's comforting domestic arts. In fact, he couldn't do without either woman. The down-to-earth, practical Ans catered to his everyday needs, while Henrietta saved him from spiritual starvation. She shared with him and Mick a fascination for the occult, and they all belonged to a circle that undertook serious research in such matters. But it was Ans who kept his household running, and so she was able to exercise virtual control over her partner, ruling out open encounters between him and Henrietta, and Vestdijk lacked the strength to challenge her.

A serious, somewhat sheltered man, Vestdijk found Henrietta an intoxicating and tantalizing presence, and he often confessed his agonies over his situation to Mick on their walks together—much to my edification, of course. Naturally I preferred the company of Henrietta to that of Ans, and just as naturally Germaine took the side of Ans. For a long time she refused to accept Henrietta: she was never very sympathetic to unfaithful husbands. But gradually Henrietta's charm and openness won her over, and she even allowed Vestdijk to bring his mistress with him on visits to us in Amsterdam—occasions Germaine tactfully refrained from mentioning to Ans.

Henrietta's own house wasn't far from ours, and when I was

about fifteen I often made a point of dropping in after school for a chat over tea and biscuits. Something she told me during one of those visits had quite an important influence on my life and career. I had just confided that I'd made up my mind to become a journalist and had already written a number of articles for my high school magazine. "Grow up, kid," she told me. "Why do you want to be called out at any odd hour to cover some boring story—some drunk knocked over in a street accident, a miserable little fire that didn't kill anybody, all the excitement of a barroom brawl? Start living your own life—do *outrageous* things *yourself* and write about them in your own books, not just grubby copy in some local rag."

I hope she was pleased with the colorful flowers that later grew from the seed she had sown in my imagination. Soon my mind was looking for the outrageous wherever I could find it. As I walked on the beach hand in hand with my father, I would imagine the comments of passersby: "Do you think that pretty girl is really his daughter, or is she some little piece of homework the old rascal has picked up?"

I was still a virgin, but I fervently hoped that was how people saw us—man and girl, lovers and proud of it.

SIMON VESTDIJK played such a major role in my father's life that their relationship intrigued me even after both of them had died. Shortly after my father's death I read in a literary journal that a man called Hans Visser was writing a biography of Vestdijk, and that he was puzzled by a lack of documentation for a crucial period in the life of this prolific writer. I wrote him and asked whether he had discovered any correspondence between Vestdijk and my father. He replied that he had indeed unearthed a mass of letters from Mick, but that he'd been unable to find any copies of the other side of a correspondence I knew had gone on between the two men from 1927 until 1960, interrupted only by the war.

I was sure there must exist a cache of these letters; my father was meticulous about his correspondence, and it was inconceivable that he wouldn't have kept such a trove of letters from his closest friend. Vestdijk was an important literary figure in Holland, and surely Mick would have expected that one day he would attract the attention of a serious biographer; these letters would be gold dust to the author. I'd never seen such letters among my father's things, but then again why would he have shown such intimate outpourings to a child? On the other hand, I thought, if any such letters existed, Germaine must have known about them. So I told her about my contact with Visser and asked whether she could shed any light on their whereabouts. But her answers were embarrassed and evasive; I sensed I was venturing on dangerous ground. But why should my mother be so sensitive about letters written so many years ago?

Gradually, the truth emerged. Through the years, Germaine confided, she had resented the intellectual bond between the two men, from which she felt excluded. Having acted for years as my father's secretary, she had the opportunity to hide Vestdijk's letters; after my father became ill she felt sure he would cease to be interested in them, perhaps even forget them altogether. Her jealousy outlived her husband: after his death she threw the entire archive into the garbage. Much as I loved my mother, I could never forgive her.

After my meeting with Visser, we two decided to publish a book of letters from Mick to Vestdijk. We met with furious opposition from Mieke, the woman Vestdijk had married after Ans's death. (His great love, Henrietta, also died not long thereafter.) His new wife, a young and devoted fan of Vestdijk, claimed ownership of the letters, but legally I owned the copyright and so was entitled to publish them. Of course, Mieke didn't know that Germaine had destroyed the other half of the correspondence, and she was terrified at what fresh scandalous stories might emerge. We had to call in a collaborator to decipher Mick's writing—a true doctor's scrawl—and some of the medical Latin he used. A mutual friend of theirs, a Dutch painter called Lucebert, illustrated the book, which

we called *A Crackling Firework*. On the cover was a photo of the
two men walking in Dam Square; the interior featured facsimiles of
some of the letters, and gazing at the familiar handwriting, I felt
almost as though I were intruding upon my father's private life. The
letters were filled with stories of his life in prewar Indonesia, and
very explicit stories of his encounters with women in Paris and the
Far East, as well as back in Holland. Knowing what I did about the
way the two men worked together, I suspected that what Mick had
written wasn't necessarily a literal account but more a piece of fantasy—a challenge to his friend to breathe life into these letters in his
own creative writing.

The publication of the book aroused considerable interest:
Vestdijk was a famous figure, and here were altogether new insights
into his character from someone who'd known him as well as anyone, including his wives and mistresses. I was invited to participate
in a series of TV programs to promote the book, and during one of
them a caller asked for my private phone number, saying that she
had something important to tell me. I called her, and a week later
she came to meet Germaine and me and tell us her story.

Our visitor was a charming, gray-haired woman, neatly and
soberly dressed, with an air of respectability. But from the photograph she brought along—showing her with Mick and his fellow
doctor Boelie—I saw that when they met she had been a beautiful
blonde in her early twenties. The three of them were standing
before a row of huts, behind which rose forbidding coils of barbed
wire. She had been an inmate of the prison camp where Mick and
Boelie had cared for hundreds of women prisoners.

Even now, so many years later, Germaine's old suspicions flared
up when she saw the picture of her dapper husband holding hands
with the attractive young woman. "My husband must have had
quite a time surrounded by all those women," she groused.

"Two handsome doctors surrounded by a couple of hundred
women," our visitor said, and then smiled. "But no, madam, it was
not the glamorous existence you might imagine. Don't forget, there

were all those kids as well, and the camps were filthy—breeding grounds for beriberi and dysentery. We were starving, and what little food we had was so unsanitary that there were always outbreaks of food poisoning." She looked at my mother earnestly. "Let me tell you what happened between me and your husband.

"One day my left arm began to swell up enormously, and a very painful sore developed near my elbow. The wound was heavily infected, and I was running a high fever. To me the sore looked cancerous, and I honestly believed I was about to die. My five-year-old son was sent to find the doctor. And Dr. Mick de Vries came to sit beside me on a rattan mat while I lay helpless in my cot." My mother's own memories must at last have been revived, for she put her arm round the woman's shoulders to comfort her as we waited for her to compose herself and continue.

"Dr. Mick sat and talked to me for hours on end to save me from drifting into a coma. He ignored the curfew, which was so strictly enforced that not even doctors were permitted to stay in the women's quarters. He called in Dr. Boelie and—communicating largely by silent gesture—the two schemed up a way to get the drugs they needed to keep me alive. Dr. Mick consulted a medical reference book that somehow he had miraculously smuggled in, and spent the night wiping the sweat from my face with a handkerchief. In the morning he cut open the wound and cleaned it out, having first hypnotized me so that I remained perfectly conscious yet unaware of any pain. The infection was so severe I was sure my arm would have to be amputated, but he made up some gauze pads out of scraps of material, and mercifully the awful pain slackened. You know, he sat with me for twenty-four hours, practically without a break."

Her cheeks were flushed; my mother gave her a cool drink, but soon our visitor was quite herself again.

"The way your husband could tell stories!" she said to Germaine. "He talked me through the night, easing my pain as if by a spell. He told Asian fairy stories, imitated the song of the birds,

and even sang some sweet Indonesian folk song—and all the time
he was stroking my arm as if to persuade the infection not to
spread."

As she paused, I asked, "So, were you charmed by my dad?"

"Of course I was; plenty of the women fancied him. But I felt
honored by him. He had saved my life, and there was no way I
could adequately thank him. But there's more to my story. A few
weeks later, when my arm was completely cured, I woke up with a
huge swelling in my leg, as if I had contracted a form of elephanti-
asis. Again I was terrified, but my little son managed to get over to
the other end of the camp, where Dr. Mick had set up a primitive
hospital with some ancient implements. He rushed over as soon as
he could, even leaving a few patients to await his return. I felt terrible having to call him out a second time. Again he saw me through
the ordeal, and this time he was able to treat me more quickly,
thanks to his supply of medication, and morphine to relieve the
pain.

" 'Doctor,' I groaned, 'I feel so weak. Do you think this time I'm
going to die?' He laughed at my panic. 'Young woman, if I didn't
let you die from that dreadful arm, why should I let you die from
something so silly as one fat leg? I won't let the angel of death carry
you off yet.' "

| |

Family and Friends?

WHEN I WAS A TEENAGER, I became increasingly aware of the growing distance between my parents. Not that there was any lack of affection, and I was as resentful as ever of their full and satisfying sex life, which remained like a beautiful garden into which I would illicitly peep from an unhappy distance. It was in their intellectual lives that Mick and Germaine diverged, and that gap grew wider as my father's friendship with Vestdijk blossomed.

In addition to his own writing, Mick found an outlet for his artistic ability and love of beauty when he became a talented weekend painter—despite being a trifle color-blind, a condition aggravated when he worked in artificial light at night. His style owed much to Monet and van Gogh; he laid the paint on thick, using his palette knife. In our house he accumulated a fine collection of art books, and in his waiting room he installed an easel so that his patients could be greeted by his vivid paintings. He donated many of his finest canvases to Vestdijk, and he in turn presented Mick with autographed first editions of his books—including a number

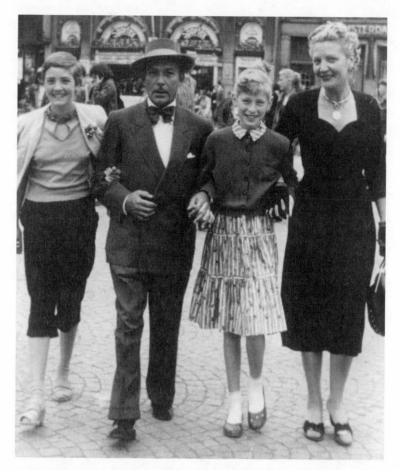

With Mick, Germaine, and my friend Dethy (second from right)

that were dedicated to Mick. Vestdijk had led the quiet life of a recluse, in stark contrast to Mick's colorful and often romantic adventures, and he was grateful to be able to transform them into works of fiction. And so Germaine suffered a double indignity: not only was she forced to play second fiddle to this other man, but she also knew with mortification that the result would be a record of her husband's infidelities, celebrated in the great man's works.

To make matters worse, Mick's passion for painting rekindled another friendship from his student days. Jan van Herwijnen was a full-time artist, and soon he was joining Mick in Vestdijk's garden, where the three of them would bask in hours of leisurely conversation—again to the exclusion of Germaine and Ans. Roaming around Amsterdam—Mick, with his dark mustache and air of brooding mystery, looking like a cross between Charlie Chaplin and Salvador Dali; Jan sporting baggy white linen trousers and brightly colored Russian shirts, his white unruly hair blowing in the wind; and Vestdijk, with slicked black hair and metal-framed glasses falling off his nose—they made quite a spectacle. Their conversations were a marvel of contrast: Vestdijk was the soul of reason and restraint, while Jan would gesticulate wildly, arguing loudly and with great animation. And Mick, Amsterdam's Don Juan, was the leader of the pack, charming both men and women wherever they went.

My mother and I sometimes accompanied my father to visit Jan at his villa in Bergen. The house's white walls were shabby, the paint flaking, and the whole place was somewhat dilapidated—but its picture windows commanded a fine view over the beach and the restless waters of the sea. And it was the chance to walk along the coast during the summer that drew my mother and me, rather than the disorder and hubbub of the house. Jan had managed to acquire four wives in his lifetime, and the racket of his brood drove Germaine to such distraction that she rarely endured it more than an hour or two before making her escape.

IF GERMAINE resented her exclusion from her husband's bohemian and intellectual adventures, she found consolation in a totally unexpected quarter—in the form of Yigal, the Russian Jew she had almost married as a teenage girl in Cologne. After leaving him practically at the altar, Germaine had long since lost track of Yigal; she knew the Nazis had confiscated his passport, and it seemed inevitable that he would have shared the fate of most other

European Jews—being herded into a cattle car and transported to the death camps in the east.

Indeed, she now learned, Yigal *had* been shipped to Auschwitz and later moved to Dachau. But there he met a strong Russian woman named Yuscha, and her support helped him to survive. As soon as they were liberated, they married and moved to Amsterdam, where all those years later Germaine came across his name by chance in the phone book. She called, they met soon after and, despite their marriages and the passing of so many years, found that the bonds of their affection were as strong as ever. Before long Yigal's wife was obliged to accept that there was another woman in her husband's life, and the old lovers went on seeing each other until Yigal's death.

After this phantom from the past returned to my mother's life, she used to take me with her on surreptitious excursions to see Yigal in the leather-goods factory he owned—visits she kept a deadly secret from Mick. I too was sworn to secrecy, recruited by Germaine as her accomplice in the conspiracy—my mother's one stand against Mick's dominance. I was fascinated at being escorted around the place by Yigal's secretary while he and Germaine were left alone and undisturbed in his office, behind discreetly closed doors. I never discovered what they were up to, but Germaine always seemed a more contented person when she emerged.

For me, the factory was a place of enchantment; for the rest of my life, the smell of leather has brought back memories of the sensuous pleasure of the rich aroma of fine leather of every conceivable shape and color all around me.

For being a good girl and keeping out of the way I was often rewarded with a belt, a purse, or a pair of sandals as we left, and Germaine would urge me not to tell Daddy where we had been. "He does not know I still see that man," she told me. "I have known him for such a long time and he is truly my best friend, someone in whom I can confide. Of course Yigal and I have no secrets, but it's best that neither his wife nor your father know about our meetings."

Young as I was, I realized there must have been some sort of love between them. And, whatever else they may have shared, I know Yigal provided my mother with a sense of her own worth. It was something she needed, a counter to the cynical or sarcastic comments she was sometimes forced to endure from Mick, and which she lacked the sense of humor to dismiss.

The rest of the time, though, I remained Mick's faithful companion—in the visits to Vestdijk, where I insisted on staying with the men, and in sharing his flirtatious fantasies on walks by ourselves. I still remember the two of us sitting on the beach or walking in a crowded street. We would gaze at passersby and rate them from one to ten on how sexy they looked. We had much the same taste, hardly ever scoring more than six or seven for Dutch men or women. When we played the same game in Italy or Spain, the scoring was much higher.

ON FRIDAY AFTERNOONS after school had finished, and often on Saturdays, my father would take a few of my school chums and me to Café Eylders on the Leidseplein. Mr. Eylders, an impressive character and a good friend of both my parents, mounted several exhibitions of my father's works in the café. Quite a few patrons expressed interest in his work, but if Mick didn't like the look of the would-be buyer, or disapproved of his character, he would refuse to sell. Inevitably close friends or members of the family acquired most of the paintings, and Vestdijk got more than anyone. After a while the walls of our own house were lined three deep with canvases.

These weekend outings turned into regular party evenings, as there were always friends at the café to join us. It was a wonderful place, with its well-worn leather sofas and boisterous card players in the corner shouting rude remarks at the passing waiters. Our big table would be covered with bowls of appetizers, nuts, and liver sausage, cheese and *bitterballen* and frequent rounds of toasted sandwiches. My mother drank modestly, medium sherry or the occasional gin and tonic, and I always had tea. Mick took soda water but also the odd glass of beer, some of which he would covertly slip to Trippie, Germaine's ubiquitous silver-gray poodle. And when it was time to go, no matter how many had joined our party uninvited, it was always Mick who picked up the tab.

By this time I was in my third year at high school, and my girlfriends were falling one after another for my dad's charms, which made me both proud and very jealous. With the passing of the years, though, my parents both seemed to be growing more mature; Germaine, now more secure in her marriage, was learning how to cope with Mick's sarcasm—and answer with her own. Life in the house on the Nassaukade grew less tense, and laughter returned to our home. And the volatile relationship between Vestdijk and Mick, which had from time to time become palpably strained, eased as they got older; they would hug and embrace like long separated lovers when they met, and radiate a golden happiness in each other's company.

12

My Heart Belongs
to Daddy

I SUPPOSE most normal kids are more attached to their mother during childhood than to the more remote figure of their father. Mother was there to cuddle them when they needed comfort, pick them up when they stumbled, and of course give them life from the milk of her breast. Only after a few years do most daughters develop a crush on their fathers.

My childhood, though, was far from normal. During the seemingly interminable time of our captivity, I was quite conscious of the presence of my mother, who risked her very life to protect me and beg or barter for the food to keep me alive, but never really knew what it was to have a father. And after our dramatic reunion, he appeared to me a magical figure who could heal our sicknesses and provide us with a home and security from a world I had good reason to regard as hostile.

The fact that Mick was a man who exuded charm, and attracted women effortlessly, must have affected me long before I was conscious of his sexuality. But as far back as I can remember, my infant

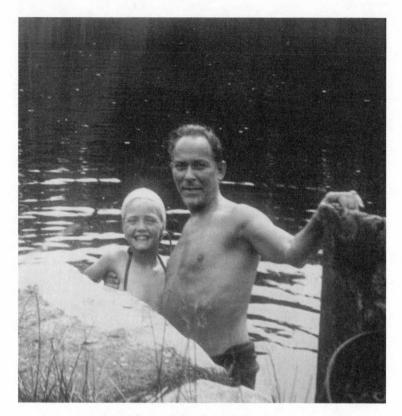

Father and daughter in the water

adulation was tinged with a precocious sensuality. I wanted to be near him—nearer than Germaine, whom I would have ousted from his affection if I had had the means. The most painful pangs of jealousy I suffered occured those nights when they made love, and I would creep out of my room to crouch on the landing outside the door of their bedroom, listening to every sound. Once I had grown out of wetting the bed, I began to wriggle into bed with my parents, always sneaking between my father and mother— bringing me closer to him than she was. If I couldn't drive my mother out of my father's bed and replace her, I was determined to join them. I think it is from those precious moments of bliss that I grew so fond of both of them, lying between the bodies of the two people I loved more than anyone else in the world. But it was only many years later, after both had died, that I understood clearly what was going on in my head in those formative nights.

Along with the bed ritual, there was also a bath ritual. Once a week, when I was very young, I would share a bath with my father. As our bodies were covered with fragrant bubbles and he soaped my doll-like body, I tingled for the first time to the caress of a man's hands, strong yet gentle. Young as I was, I remember being curious about that odd part of his body; it was my first glimpse of a male sex organ. Yet in truth I wasn't all that precocious and was actually more intrigued by his hands as they played water games or created shadow plays on the wall.

If my childish ambition to supplant my mother was to be fulfilled, I realized, I'd have to impress my father with my achievements. My school reports were unlikely to dazzle him, but music was a more promising arena. Germaine was fond of music, but she didn't play an instrument—so here was a natural opportunity to shine. At the age of seven I started taking piano lessons from Maurice Agsteribbe, an Auschwitz survivor, who tried to inculcate in me his own reverence for the works of Bach and inspire me to tackle the preludes and fugues of the *Well-Tempered Clavier*. My own tastes ran more to the likes of Georges Moustaki, Jacques Brel, or Juliette Greco, Pete Seeger and Frank Sinatra. But to please my father I needed to excel in the classical world, and I cultivated a taste for the austerity of the *Trois Gymnopédies* of Erik Satie and the elusive impressionism of Albéniz. Indeed, by the time I was twelve I was doing well enough at the keyboard to win a few competitions, which pleased my father no end.

My instructor, Maurice—Maupie, as we called him—was a poor soul who lived a quiet and lonely life. I still remember him, always in the same coffee-stained sweater, once black but now gray with grime, his unruly shock of hair the same dingy shade, in dramatic contrast with his pitch-black eyebrows. Maupie possessed one uncanny knack: during my lessons he would gently nod off and start to snore, apparently oblivious to my efforts at the keyboard, his multiple chins resting peacefully on his chest as he slumbered while I struggled with Satie. But as soon as I struck a wrong note he would correct me without even opening his eyes. And when my mother came into the room with coffee he was instantly awake, eyes wide open and humming along happily with whatever I was playing.

Maupie, I learned later, was haunted by the memory of an overwhelming tragedy. During the Nazi occupation his only son had gone into hiding, and one summer night Maupie risked visiting him. The youth concealed himself on a window seat behind a thick, black curtain to hide from visitors who couldn't be trusted. That night he was sitting there behind the curtain, chatting with his father, when Maupie made a joke and his son rocked with laughter. The window behind him was usually shut, but this was such a hot day that it was open, and when the boy leaned against the curtain he fell and crashed to his death on the pavement below. His father was destroyed by grief and guilt—the boy had died because of something he had said.

He must have felt it was a judgment when, two days later, he was rounded up by the Gestapo and loaded into a filthy cattle car, destination Auschwitz.

The tragedies of his own life and of his son's death were blows from which Maupie never recovered. He became more and more depressed, a recluse, watched over only by his cat, whose matted fur mirrored his master's own unkempt locks. His home was dingy and unswept, and barely furnished apart from three majestic grand pianos: when he finally died at the age of sixty-eight, it was days before a neighbor discovered the dead man and the starving cat on New Year's Eve. He had no girlfriend or boyfriend; his sole passion was music—particularly that of Beethoven, to whom he bore a striking resemblance.

Even as a child I sensed something odd about Maupie—something more than the sadness of his son's story. But it was not until some years later that Germaine felt I was old enough to hear the truth. "That poor man!" she told me. "He was subjected to the most barbaric medical experiments in that death camp."

And then, lowering her voice as if in respect, she whispered: "Then they castrated him."

THE OTHER MUSICAL INFLUENCE on my childhood was that of my Uncle Julius. Another survivor of the Indonesian prison camps, he was not actually related but was so close a friend of my parents that he was Uncle Julius to me. Just as Maupie's only soul mate was his piano, Julius was wedded to his cello. A gentle yet lively little man, as leader of the cello section of the Concertgebouw Orchestra he had played under the baton of the greatest conductors of his day. He also directed a string quartet, specializing in romantic pieces they would play in such venues as hospitals. Perhaps it was to delight Germaine that he performed extracts from Viennese operettas in our house, but it was his soulful playing of Max Bruch's arrangement of *Kol Nidrei*, the poignant elegy that introduces the Jewish Day of Atonement, that always reduced my father and me to tears. My own appreciation of great music was certainly nurtured by those two dear old men, but I must admit there were some concerts where my attention wandered, and I would cast my eye over the orchestra and fantasize having a romance with the most attractive instrumentalist. But such moments remained mere childish daydreams. At that stage in my life, all my sexual feelings were concentrated on my father, and my ambition to outdo Germaine.

EVEN BEFORE reaching puberty, I felt the need for company in bed. So on those nights when I failed to insinuate myself between my parents, I would console myself by sleeping with a pillow—known as a *gooling* in Indonesia—firmly between my legs, a habit I maintain to this day. It isn't much of a substitute for a man, but this "Dutch wife" provides a shred of comfort and some relief from the dread of sleeping alone in the dark, the phobia that has haunted me since my childhood in the camp.

Despite my early experiences of sexual arousal, physically I was a late developer, not menstruating until I was thirteen. Only a few years later, though, I already appeared more mature than I was. I went out with a boy named Roger when I was twelve; we never got beyond innocent fondling, but Germaine already suspected I was carrying on behind her back, deceiving my parents and becoming, in her eyes, depraved. She started prying into how I spent my time, and her case against me was clinched after she broke the lock on my private diary—and read there all the intimate fantasies and confidences of a teenage girl.

With puberty I had begun suffering from that dreadful feeling of loneliness when one is no longer a child but not yet accepted as an adult; to ease the pain I took refuge in my diary, which I started keeping when I was eleven, and now filled several discreetly locked notebooks. But it was when I was nearly sixteen and met Daantje, my first true boyfriend, that the entries had become intimate—and, to my mother, shocking. I even named my diary (Danny); there I recorded my fears and sadness over fights between my parents, my hopes for the future, and my desire to break free, travel the world, and have a life of my own. I described how, when no more than a child, I had played on our porch with an equally innocent little boy the age-old games of nurses-and-doctors and I'll-show-you-mine-if-you-show-me-yours.

But I also wrote about my sexual escapades with Daantje, in the Beatrix Park or on the sand dunes behind the beach. I described the many voyeurs we encountered, lying in the grass and peeping at us as we kissed and cuddled and felt each other's bodies. Many were the packets of cigarettes with which we bribed the park atten-

dants, patrolling with their vicious Dobermans, not to report us to
school—or, worse, to our parents for "indecent exposure." Yet I
always bore in mind my mother's warning to retain my virginity—
or, I well believed, my husband would regard me as no more than
a whore, a slut. And so I was still a virgin when my mother rifled
my diary while I was away for a week on a school trip.

When I got home, exhausted but happy and bursting to tell her
all about what had happened during my week away, she shut me up
and informed me sternly that in the morning she and my father
would confront me about some very serious matters. She refused to
say more and left me fearful but angry that she'd shown no interest
in my first trip away from home. My father and mother had always
been very strict, even overprotective, never allowing me to stay out
later than half past ten, and until this trip, being away overnight
was absolutely forbidden.

That night I slept badly, worrying what I could possibly have
done to anger my mother. I tossed and turned, and when I did fall
into a fitful sleep the old nightmares returned: the savage faces of
the Japanese soldiers, shrieking and menacing me in my slumber;
women and children beaten and bleeding; and through it all I
heard the voice of my mother screaming in torture. When I awoke,
I had once more soaked the bed.

Ashamed, I slunk out of my bedroom and apologized for my
relapse. My mother's tone was unsympathetic. "Hurry into the bath
and clean yourself up. Then come straight into our bedroom." My
only consolation was that the whole affair was clearly so urgent that
I was spared the mushy porridge that was my regular breakfast.

I slipped on my baby-doll nightdress and crept into the bedroom, where my father was seated in a fauteuil beside the bed,
wearing one of his beautiful Chinese black silk kimonos decorated
with red, yellow, and green dragons, fastened loosely by a black
belt. He looked stern, but oh so handsome! Before he could utter
a word, my mother produced with a flourish poor Danny Diary,
tore it open, the pages looking like the legs of a spread-eagled baby.

Before my horrified eyes, she ripped the pages out and hurled them into the fireplace. Then she threw some alcohol and a lighted match onto them, and they burst into flames.

I shall never forget the trauma of the sound of the pages of my life being torn to shreds. Years later, when I was signing copies of *The Happy Hooker* in a bookstore in front of Philadelphia's Penn Station, a burly man in overalls strode up with a scowl on his face and without saying a word tore one of the books to pieces. He went on shredding the fragments until the book was little more than a scattering of confetti. At that moment, just as I had while standing before my furious mother, I felt a sense of profound desecration. The book had taken nine months of my life, as had Danny Diary; it was as though these vandals were murdering a child to whom I had given birth.

I begged Germaine to stop. I had so little private life—why must it be so pitilessly destroyed?

"You filthy little slut! This will teach you not to confide secrets on paper in this house. Nothing is sacrosanct in our home, and you have no right to keep secrets from your parents. Do you understand? Remember that I am your mother. You are to listen to me and respect me. How dare you write insulting and wicked things about me in that filthy diary of yours? How could you write how much you hated me for yelling at your father? Don't you understand that he deserved everything I said? You are like him—both of you misbehave. I must have *honesty*! So tell me, why did you have to play around with that boy? What's going on between you and Daantje? I knew you were up to no good, always going out on his scooter to the Amsterdamse Bos, or the Beatrix Park. Disgusting!"

She was screaming hysterically, completely out of control—yet I thought she looked radiant, alive, and very sexy. Usually it was my dad who staged the virtuoso performances in our house; all I could think was, Go for it, Mom—kill two birds with one stone and give

Daddy hell as well. I'd never seen her so angry, though Mick sat as calm and silent as a brooding Buddha.

Germaine wheeled on him. "Mick, will you do something about your child? She really is your daughter; each of you is as bad as the other. Don't just sit there saying nothing. Both of you have those stupid poker faces. She could do with a good thrashing. You cannot expect me to hit my own child. Be a man and give her the spanking she deserves."

My father had never until that moment raised his hand against me. Now, without saying a word, he submitted to his wife's demand. He looked miserable at having to act against his heart, but I felt a flare of excitement nevertheless as I spread my thinly clad body on his lap, much higher than over his knees as Germaine expected. Standing by the door, she shouted: "*Now*, Mick, hit her! Hit her now!"

On that word, his hand crashed down on my ass. I never suspected he had such strength. It hurt like a knife biting into my bare flesh. But each time he struck, my body thrust harder into his groin, and I could sense his own excitement rising. To this day, I remember the feel of his silk gown and the musky smell of his sweat as he got more and more worked up at each smack on my buttocks. As for me, I felt as if he were hitting that same spot his fingers had brushed by when he had operated on me in the concentration camp—an area that was growing warmer and harder now with every blow. My whole body glowed—my buttocks must by then have been fiery red—but I was becoming consumed by passion. My screams grew more intense, my movements spasmodic, and at that moment I believe I experienced the first shattering orgasm of my life. I felt that this could go on forever, but Germaine must have realized that things were getting out of hand.

"Stop it, Mick," she cried. "You're hitting her too hard. That's enough!"

"No, I deserve it, go on!" I wasn't finished yet.

Mick must have understood what was happening to me. Instead of stopping immediately, he gradually slackened the violence and frequency of his smacks until my body ceased shuddering. Then he held me in his arms for a few moments and hugged me before standing up and straightening his kimono to conceal his own arousal. The incident was never mentioned again; it remained a secret shared by our family triangle. But it was after this episode that I stopped sleeping in my parents' bed. The uncomplicated life of childhood had gone forever, and I simply wasn't sure I could control what might happen if I became aroused in the night. Everything had changed.

IN THE WEEKS and months that followed, Germaine's attitude hardened. She became even more stern and watchful of my conduct. Above all, her jealousy of my closeness to my father grew more intense. They continued to be a loving couple, though, and that in turn only increased my own unhappiness. My parents had never been uneasy about walking around in the house without clothes, and I was accustomed to the sight of their naked bodies. Now all it would take was for my father to kiss his wife lovingly on her forehead or cheek, or stride up behind her and wrap his arms around her shoulders, and I would run out of the room to be spared the sight of their affection. How much more I resented it when they emerged together from a prolonged visit to their bedroom or bathroom, my father radiating happiness, my mother smiling with unaccustomed coyness, sexy and satisfied. They were great flirts, both of them, right until my father's final illness.

The time had come for me to find my own sexual fulfillment, outside the loves and jealousies of my family.

13

From First Lust to
First Love

BEFORE THAT ILL-FATED school trip, I had always accompanied my parents on holiday. My father's favorite expeditions were to the mountains of Austria or Switzerland, where we would hike for hours, my father out front with his hand-carved walking stick.

My own preference was for the Italian lakes or the coast, where I could laze on a beach and soak up the sun. That also suited Germaine; much to the annoyance of my father, she would flirt mildly with gallant young tennis coaches, who just had to hold her hand to show her a more effective grip—of her racket, of course. While she played doubles with other sporty guests, her husband preferred to sit under a tree, reading, composing a poem, writing, or simply meditating.

When I was twelve my parents took me to Germany, where we stayed at a pension not far from a big farm. With my tomboy looks I was instantly accepted by the male population of the village—and especially by one big, blond farmhand with great rippling muscles. Rudolf was as handsome as a young god, at least in my eyes, and I was intoxicated by the heavy, sweaty smell of his body. He would place me on the seat in front of him and take me for rides on his motorbike; breathing down my neck, he pressed my shoulders tight against him, and sometimes let his hand stray over my nascent breasts.

Some days Rudolf would come back with me for a bite of lunch, and it seemed to me that Germaine was as much attracted to him as I was. Was it just my imagination that she would spray herself with her most seductive perfume when she knew my friend was coming? And one time, when my father was away, Rudolf emerged from our bathroom wearing only a skimpy towel, his tanned body displayed as if for our admiration. As she handed him a cold beer, my mother's hand brushed against his bare shoulder. I saw her blush, which only fired my own newly aroused imagination: I convinced myself—quite unjustifiably—that if I hadn't been present, my own mother would have succumbed to Rudolf's animal attraction. Again I had set myself up as her rival: no way would I be her accomplice in deceiving my father.

I was so jealous that I resolved the following day that Rudolf and I should drive a few miles down the road and stop near a highly convenient haystack for a good wrestle. I tossed with him, inhaling his strong aroma, pushing my body hard against his, grabbing his flesh, tugging his T-shirt out of his jeans, exploring his belly button and letting my hands wander over his hairy body. I pushed my tongue into his ear and delicately kissed his earlobe. Soon I could tell that Rudolf was aroused; having dismounted from the bike, he set his mind to mounting me. When he managed to thrust his tongue deep inside my mouth, I began to get scared; the heat of his body radiated through my flimsy summer dress, and my white cotton knickers were wet with my excitement. There was a wild gleam in his eyes, and his breathing sounded ragged. He grasped my hand and thrust it between his legs, and I knew from the bulge in his jeans that what had started as a harmless game of wrestling was about to turn into something more serious. My mother's words

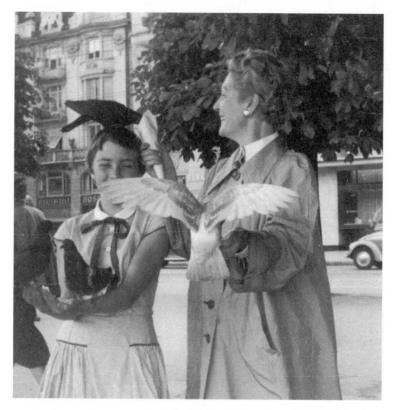

On vacation in Italy

echoed in my mind—make sure you marry as a virgin, and never let a man undress you until you're old enough to know you are truly in love. Much as I liked Rudolf, I certainly knew I wasn't in love with him. He was strong as an ox, and I had a hell of a struggle breaking free: one of my sandals and a shoulder strap were broken before he agreed not to molest me further.

After we cooled down, we shared a lunch of salami sandwiches and apples. Then he offered to take me back to the farm slaughterhouse and show me the pigs and calves being prepared for the butcher. I was grateful to have an outlet for the adrenaline that was pumping through my body, and after watching the livestock being killed, the two of us joined the cook drowning some newborn kittens—much to my parents' horror when we shared the story later. As a trophy I brought home the eye of a freshly killed calf, and described in terrible detail the way I had spent the second half of the afternoon. (It seemed wise not to describe the first.) My poor father abhorred cruelty toward animals, so I must have caused him some real pain that afternoon.

On another occasion, I came across a snake while walking along a mountain path. Before my father could stop me I attacked it with a stick, killing it instantly.

"Now what do you think you've achieved?" he asked. "Don't you know snakes live as couples, just as we do? Its mate is sure to come looking for it, and she'll be sorely disappointed." Sure enough, the next morning I nearly trod on the snake's mate—but this time I left it alone.

I never attained that gentleness that was so strong a quality in the character of my father, but I did try to acquire something of his wisdom. Every morning, even after one of my sadistic outbursts, I would enjoy the tranquillity of a family breakfast on the terrace, eating pieces of Toblerone chocolate spread on fresh croissants or baguettes. My father would talk about the book he was reading while Germaine related all the village gossip. What a contrast!

THE DANNY DIARY EPISODE was a turning point in my development and my parents' attitude toward me. I'd grown up in a relaxed, open-minded home without any trace of shame in our bodies. We had always shown our love and affection for one another without embarrassment; there was a lot of kissing and hugging and holding, especially between my dad and me, but my mom hugged and kissed me too: many times the three of us were naked in the bathroom together, my father taking a shower or shaving, my mother and I sitting with him and talking, covered only by a towel or a sarong.

But our bathroom rituals had stopped when I was thirteen and my mom discovered I was growing body hair, and that my breasts had begun to swell. I can appreciate now that my mother's outrage over my diary entries was an expression of her concern—and of the overprotectiveness so often fostered by the cruelties of wartime. She became obsessed that I should be spared any future unhappiness—and as a result I developed into a moody teenager, a loner at school, and was left much to my own devices.

So I became one of those pale-faced, androgynous kids who hung out in arty little cafés near school, sipping hot chocolate with whipped cream or a fancy flavored tea. In that age of innocence before hash cafés, when *coke* meant cola and pills were for headaches, we found our cool in the music of Dave Brubeck and Miles Davis, Sidney Bechet and Louis Armstrong, and the soulful blues of Ella Fitzgerald and Bessie Smith. But what really got to us were those sad, sad stories in the heart-rending voice of Billie Holiday. I had become more introverted, withdrawing into my room—a sanctum for my teenage dreams and fantasies, but also a refuge from the angry words my mom would occasionally hurl at my father over some new peccadillo. I plastered the walls with posters, which I changed every few months: Marlon Brando, Brigitte Bardot, Claudia Cardinale, Kirk Douglas, Lauren Bacall, and James Dean. Peggy Lee was on my turntable at home, but my heart belonged to Charles Aznavour, whose voice mesmerized me and with whom I had fallen madly in love.

By sixteen I'd begun to feel more comfortable about becoming a woman, and I gradually grew more outgoing, almost extroverted. At school I got into all sorts of mischief, wrote songs for the school cabaret, became the editor of the school paper, wrote lots of short stories, and fell hopelessly in love with a real flesh-and-blood boy, not some remote pop idol.

At home I'd tried to compete with my mother for my father's affection, but I didn't have her elegant long legs, nor could I walk for hours in high heels. I certainly didn't have her exquisite taste in clothes and accessories, but I was fascinated by her sexy, long gowns, short lacy slips with little matching corselets, bras and panties in different colors, and exquisite, fine stockings.

"Vera," she would lecture me, "when you grow up you'll wear this kind of underwear too. Just always make sure your husband never sees you wearing any other kind. And lingerie lying over the back of a chair, or dropped carelessly about, loses all its appeal. Always put it away neatly before you go to bed, out of your husband's sight, to preserve its air of mystery. It's one of those things men really appreciate."

14

Eroticism at
the Barlaeus Gymnasium

WHEN I TURNED FIFTEEN, I still had that boyishness about me. When I walked the street that summer in my shorts and black sweater—especially if I'd just been swimming and my short hair was wet—sometimes a butcher boy making deliveries on his bike would actually stop to stare and call out, "Hey, you—are you a boy or a girl?"

One reason I seemed so boyish, of course, was my flat chest. For years I'd had an inferiority complex about my waiflike look . . . that is, until I met Eric, or "Puck," as most of our classmates called him after he took a convincing turn in the role in *A Midsummer Night's Dream* on our school stage.

I preferred "Eric": it sounded more masculine, and that he surely was, especially compared with the pimply-faced kids in my class. He must have been eighteen, and he was quite a character: thick, unruly pitch-black hair that curled shoulder length around his pale face, the brightest of blue eyes surrounded by dark, long eyelashes, a nose big and bent, and a prominent chin that made him look rebellious and strong. He was handsome in a rugged way and had something of the ape about him, especially as his chest was covered with black hair.

Eric had left school to join the merchant navy when he was very young; then after traveling the world for a few years he returned to finish high school at the Barlaeus Gymnasium, where we met. At school he started acting in the student cabaret and soon discovered his niche as an aspiring stage actor. As soon as he finished high school he enrolled at the Amsterdam Theater School and began writing plays and sketches. Girls of my age as well as his all fell for Eric's charm and worldly attitude: he was secure, mature, and most of all, strong—though he could also be strong-willed and temperamental, even moody. He could have had any woman at his fingertips, but for some miraculous reason he seemed to have eyes for only me. Soon we were going steady and shared almost every moment of our spare time.

Eric's father had died in Auschwitz; like me an only child, he had a tough mother who often made life hell for him. For me this totally new experience—being in love with a man other than my father—was also a way to leave my parents to themselves and escape the stifling grip of my mother. Even at sixteen I still had to be home every night by eleven, and wearing any kind of makeup was forbidden.

My father took an instant liking to Eric—they were avid readers with similar tastes—and my parents often came to the school cabarets; when my father watched Eric do Charlie Chaplin's routine with the flower, he was won over for good. Germaine was equally disarmed by Eric's wit and charming behavior, though given our age difference and Eric's wild years on the seas, she was soon worrying about her daughter's virginity. Nowadays I know mothers who can't be bothered to inform their daughters about sexual education, simply giving them a box of birth-control pills the moment they start dating; often the girls themselves reject the offer, preferring to decide themselves when the time is right. My mother was far from liberated; if anything she was too protective toward her baby chick. In our house there were no major lessons about sex; instead, medical books started showing up on our coffee tables featuring horrible pictures of what could happen to people if they had sex: gonorrhea, syphilis, children born with half-noses or cleft palates—you name it! When I asked Eric one day why he never fancied the older girls who swarmed around him like bees—and who obviously weren't virgins—he shrugged his broad shoulders. "Your mom has nothing to worry about. I only love you more for your purity and innocence, your giddiness and enthusiasm—and because you always laugh at the right moment when I say something funny, even when others don't seem to get it." Then, from out of nowhere, he produced a rose.

One day, in the very early stages of our romance, we visited the Atomium, a vast exhibition space swarming with thousands of people. We were walking with our bikes, but we were paying so much attention to each other that our handlebars kept getting tangled, so we placed them against a tree and locked them together with one big chain. Standing still in a quiet, shady spot, we held each other for an eternity against one of the big comforting trees. Eric caressed my face, stroked my short hair, kissed my earlobe, then touched my eyelids with his mouth ever so softly. Finally his full lips pressed gently against mine. Oh, how I loved the way he kissed me then! I'd never really been kissed by anyone before, and I loved the way he pressed his closed lips first gently, then more firmly, onto mine. As we closed our eyes and his hands held mine, his body pushed closely against me; I could feel the hair on his chest tickle my upper arm.

He never kissed me like every other man who would follow— their mouths open, long, wet tongues shoving deep inside my throat. Eric's kisses were moist, intense, and innocent. I loved to inhale the rising odor of his body as he grew excited; one day, when he wasn't looking, I stole the red T-shirt he used to wear onstage and kept it to remind me of his scent when he wasn't around.

Our love affair was utterly pure and remained that way, which surprises me even today. Later, as the months went by, he started exploring my body; as I relaxed beside him on the beach in a bikini, his hands would move from the nape of my neck down my back to

my thighs, and I could feel the thrill down my spine and in the rosy
tips of my breasts. Yet we never saw each other naked: little Vera
remained pure, just as Germaine had ordered.

Still, I wasn't so innocent that I never dreamed of bigger
things—specifically, bigger breasts. Being three years Eric's junior
and still a virgin was enough to give me a bit of an inferiority complex, but it was my flat chest that really bothered me: I pined for a
figure like my mother's, but somehow my body seemed determined
not to grow where I needed it. So I decided to help nature out a bit.
As soon as I'd made it a few streets away from home on my bike
every morning, I'd stop and take off the white socks I wore with my
pink queenies. The style in those days was the style everyone
remembers from *American Graffiti:* big full petticoats, black-and-
white check skirts, Lana Turner–type tight sweaters with a waistline
like a wasp, and a broad belt. After I'd made sure there was no one
else around, I'd cram the socks inside my bra one after the other,
arrange them so they looked natural, and then went on to school,
stacked as nicely as the luckiest of my girlfriends.

On the way home, of course, I would reverse the procedure. But
one day, as I was hurrying home with a girlfriend, I forgot all about
them. My mother took one look at me and said in mock surprise:
"Well, you certainly have become a woman overnight, haven't
you?" Fortunately my girlfriend had already left, sparing me at least
a modicum of embarrassment.

One night, after watching Eric perform at the cabaret, followed
by an evening of dancing, I was walking hand in hand with him
down the school corridor. As usual, a few jealous girls smiled and
stopped to compliment him on his performance—but this time I
noticed a few of them looking at me oddly as I walked past. I
couldn't figure out what was wrong until my friend Annemarie
took me aside, out of Eric's earshot.

"You know, your one tit seems to be much bigger than the
other. You're not wearing *padding* or anything, are you?"

I don't blush easily, but that evening I was glowing like a siren.

I ran to the bathroom to remove the other sock, and swore then and there to get out of the fake-tit business for good. As if as a reward, a few months later Mother Nature chipped in and brought me just what I'd been waiting for.

The respect and adoration Eric showed never diminished, though when he left school again after his final exams somehow our relationship came to an abrupt end. After our platonic affair ended I finally gave myself to another boy: Daantje, blond, blue-eyed, straight hair, more Dutch than you could imagine, artistic and funny, with a cheerful disposition. After a year of romance, sneaking out to parks or beaches to get close, he deflowered me in a perfect manner. I had obeyed my mother's words—"Child, do marry as a virgin"—for seventeen and a half years; Daantje was no great love, but he'd been a friend for years, and I decided to wait no more.

Still, I look back now with gratitude that I kept my childish innocence while Eric and I were dating; I would hate to have missed Eric's protectiveness, the fatherly side of his nature. Not to mention the entertainment value he brought to my teenage life: I still remember the wild stories Eric used to tell me about being at sea, fighting high waves, or about his visits to strange shores, scouting out bars and brothels with his fellow sailors. It was never quite clear to me whether he went to hookers or not; he wisely left that unsaid, and I never asked.

ABOUT TWENTY-FIVE YEARS LATER, after my own travels around the world, I too returned to the safe haven of Amsterdam— and before long I was sitting in a half-empty theater, watching Eric in performance. Physically, he hadn't changed much: he had the same rugged features and strong chin, hair still thick and unruly, though beginning to gray, and there were some lines around his eyes. When I went backstage he greeted me with a great hug; there was still the same warmth, that spark between us. I was no longer the innocent schoolgirl, but I felt something of my lost youth, as if a purer blood were suddenly running through my veins.

We went back to my house and talked until the sun rose. His wife had left him to live with another woman, informing him that she'd never loved him and had married him only in order to have a child. Worse yet, he told me, he found no special fulfillment in his profession; for a time he'd belonged to an established theater group, which gave him a regular income, but his colleagues found him impossible, because of his emotional state, and he was thrown out. Reduced to the uncertain life of a freelance performer, he eked out a living washing dishes in a busy Turkish restaurant. Spending evenings playing chess at a local club was his only diversion.

He had given up women after the breakup of his marriage, he told me, but nevertheless we ended up in bed—our first time together, after a quarter of a century. I was not disappointed. He was a wonderful lover, big and strong, his tender touch intact—and yet I noticed that his body had not been used for a long time. Now his dry skin came to life under my agile fingers; I caressed him, pulled him by his hair, even bit him gently on his nipples. Finally we were able to let go of all our emotions and do what we had always wanted to do, even as children.

Our love affair carried on sporadically for half a year or so, but not forever. The same warmth still went through our bodies when we met and made love, but in his eyes I could see a bitter disappointment with the world, and with himself, that upset me too much. At school Eric had played the lead in Molière's *The Misanthrope;* now he seemed to have adopted the character in real life. He still treated me with the greatest respect, but his old rebellious, recalcitrant attitude darkened our time together. When we made love it was often with the Beatles in the background, bringing back memories of our youth; now I made him a present of the White Album, and went on my way once again.

Not long after we'd parted again, Eric died suddenly, his fifteen-year-old daughter at his side. It was called a heart attack, but it was clear to me that what really killed Eric was being lonely, misunderstood, and miserable.

Before he was buried, friends were invited to say their farewells at an open-casket wake. I decided to tell my mother about his death, and though she'd never completely trusted him—she still believed he'd deflowered me years ago—she agreed reluctantly to accompany me as I paid my last respects.

There he was: our Puck, my Eric. The Turkish restaurant had taken out a big advertisement in the local paper saluting him as the best dishwasher they had ever had, and announcing that they would be closing the restaurant the day of his funeral. The chess club he'd belonged to for fifteen years also placed a small ad, declaring that they'd lost an excellent, though challenging, mate as a chess player, and that everybody would miss him.

Eric was dressed in his usual black sweater, surrounded by dozens of bouquets of flowers, and by fellow students from our days at the Barlaeus Gymnasium. He'd obviously made an impact on many more people than he had ever dreamed of seeing again in his life. Difficult though he may have been, he was always charismatic.

But something was wrong with the sight of our old Puck, this man I used to love so much. Many who knew him left the casket wearing puzzled looks, but I knew it as soon as I looked at his face. Of course he'd been made up; there was nothing to be done about that, of course. But what else had the mortician done? It was his hair! It was still thick, though now totally gray—but someone had combed it all neatly back behind his ears, as if he'd been a businessman.

"This isn't the man we all knew," I said. My classmates nodded in agreement.

"This is not our Puck," I repeated softly as I leaned over the coffin and gently touched his ice-cold forehead. It was the first time I'd ever touched the skin of a dead person, like marble beneath my fingers. I touched his cheek with the back of my hand, then slowly took his hair between my fingers, committing its texture to memory. I pulled it from behind his ears, then messed it up a bit until it was as wild and unruly as he wore it in life.

"There, that's our Puck again," someone said.

15

Doctor No More

ONE OF THE MOST vivid memories of my childhood was of watching my parents together. I had grown accustomed to my parents' love for each other, though at first I was envious and resentful that I was being excluded from something so wonderful and exciting: my father standing behind my mother as she stood before the bathroom basin, his arms around her, the two of them transfixed in ecstasy for what seemed to me a lifetime, motionless and completely absorbed in each other. But it was through seeing them together in the kitchen that I came to appreciate the coyly seductive way my mother moved, inviting the same response from her mate as she had in the bathroom.

My dad would do anything to be near his wife, even when he had to work. He would find an opportunity to slip into the living room, which adjoined his doctor's office, embrace her, and stroke her hair. He was so attentive, complimenting her dress or admiring the way she looked. And he had a routine I loved to watch: lighting a cigarette and transferring it from his mouth to my mom's before lighting another for himself. He would rarely have time to finish his cigarette, leaving it smoldering in the ashtray as he hurried back to his practice, but it was one more stolen moment together. Even in front of his patients, if my mother came in and smiled at him he would melt and let his fingers brush against her. The patients never objected; better a contented and satisfied doctor, I suppose, than one who was morose and irritable.

And even despite my jealousy, the days when they made love were still the highlights of my childhood—both because I was swept up in their happiness and because before the day was out I usually got some treat: a shopping spree, a trip to the movies, an extra helping of a favorite dessert.

TO HIS FRIENDS, Mick must have appeared to be enjoying all the fruits of success and happiness. He had such a positive view of life, caring for those sick in body or mind while devoting much of his time to his artistic side through painting and prose. On top of that, he had the satisfaction of knowing how attractive he was to women, and I know he savored the occasional succulent forbidden fruit while maintaining a stable and fulfilled family life. Even after the expulsion of the mink-clad mustard maid, from time to time Germaine lost her temper over his extramarital activities. One morning in the heat of midsummer, for instance, she noticed that he'd been keeping his pajama shirt or bathrobe on while shaving in the morning. So she strode into the bathroom, taking him by surprise, and ripped off his jacket, revealing four long scarlet scratches. There was no way the scars could be blamed on Jessica, our well-behaved cat; the pussy who'd left her mark on Mick's body undoubtedly had two legs. For several days afterward he was in the doghouse; yet after such outbursts their love and pleasure in each other's bodies seemed to grow even more intense.

As I grew older, I found a new source of delight in my own shared intimacies with him. We still had our walks on the beach together, and when I became a teenager our conversations turned to literature and the arts. During our family's occasional weekend outings in Paris, he shared his enthusiasm for chanteuses like Edith Piaf, and I discovered the works of Jean-Paul Sartre and Simone de Beauvoir—which in turn rekindled my interest in the writings of Vestdijk, and of course in my father himself.

Yet there was a darker side to my father's life, which would eventually eclipse all else. Like so many prison-camp survivors, he continued to suffer from the brutal mistreatment he had endured. He suffered pains in his neck and back, and as the years passed they became ever more severe. Patients who came to him with their aches and pains never suspected for a moment that their doctor was injecting himself with powerful painkillers. He allowed no one else to administer the injections, since they had to be placed with the utmost precision; a mere millimeter misjudgment might have meant permanent paralysis. Yet my father's pain also afforded me a chance to repay in some measure the love and kindness he had shown me: I found that I had a natural gift for massage, and he eventually came to welcome the long, deep massages that penetrated his taut muscles and the damaged joints of his spine, and the reprieve from agony I was able to bring him.

At the same time, the relentless strain of his work was taking its toll. He sought relief, spending more and more of his free time indulging his passion for painting. But after a while Germaine forbid him to continue filling the house with canvases, and in his depressed state he took the rejection hard. Suddenly he was no longer the dashing, youthful Dr. Don Juan; his eyes, once so bright, became dull, and his thick black hair grew thin and gray. His hairline receded; his cheeks began to look sunken, his forehead bare and pronounced. I believe he was suffering a genuine emotional and physical breakdown; his appetite disappeared, and he withdrew into his one true pleasure: the inner world of literature. Worried by his low spirits and general listlessness, Germaine summoned my Uncle Julius, so cheerful and friendly that he could generally dispel any depression. But not this time. I could see my beloved father going to pieces before my eyes.

Regardless of his own health, of course, there was an unending list of patients clamoring for his attention, and the combination of daily consultations and house calls took its toll. When he wasn't painfully climbing the steep, rickety staircases of old canal houses, he was often obliged to clamber aboard houseboats, against the rain and snow of the bleak Dutch winters. On one such winter night he slipped off the gangplank and plunged into the freezing water. My father had never learned to swim, and he was panic-stricken until a nearby skipper hauled him aboard.

While he still rejoiced in his skills as a healer, the drudgery of general practice held no charm for my father, and the shock of this close encounter forced him to lighten his workload. He cut back his practice by half. But within six months he saw that half-measures wouldn't suffice. The time had come to quit. Within weeks he'd sold the practice—and our home along with it—to a young Indonesian doctor; it went for a song, but the relief from obligation was all my father was looking for. The new man had none of Mick's vibrant character, but he had the decency to allow us to store some of our possessions in the basement while we found somewhere new to live.

FOR YEARS Mick had suffered from high blood pressure, but he had generally been healthy enough to look forward to an enjoyable retirement. Hoping that some relaxation in the sun far away from the gloom of another Amsterdam winter would help restore him, we moved to Valencia, Spain. The affectionate farewell we received from friends and former patients was so heartfelt that my parents were in tears at the good-bye party they gave. In their generosity they even took up a collection that provided us with the money we needed to move to our new country.

At first Mick benefited from the change of environment, and within weeks he was making his way with reasonable fluency in Spanish. His mood lightened; his appetite returned, and he lost that deathly pallor. But this remission would be short-lived; he suffered his first stroke in Valencia—a mild one, to be sure, but enough to leave his face partially paralyzed and his spirits dampened.

I had finished high school, gratifying my father by graduating with top marks. Eager to be independent, I decided not to continue my studies and took a job as a secretary. But the work was dull, and there was clearly no future for an ambitious teenager in the firm. So when Manpower, the temporary employment agency, announced a competition for the best secretary in Holland, with a prize of a thousand dollars, television interviews, magazine articles, and a trip to England, I went for it with all guns blazing! For two months competitors all over Holland battled it out, but I was determined to win.

In Valencia I received a letter informing me that I'd made it through the preliminary round, and asking me to return to Amsterdam for the contest finals and the presentation ceremony. My parents wanted to be there for support, and despite being in Spain my father's ill health persisted, so my parents resolved to return to Amsterdam for good, bringing our short Valencia interlude to a close. As if by a miracle, we learned that a former colleague of Mick's in his days as a ship's doctor had died, and his widow was happy to give us their apartment, now too large for her. Another piece in the jigsaw of our life had fallen into place, and there we were, back in Amsterdam.

I won the competition; more important than the prizes and publicity, though, was the satisfaction of seeing my father so proud of me. He must have been amused at my adroitness in mentioning the name of Manpower no less than eight times in one TV interview. The company was so impressed that they immediately hired me to manage a unit at their head office, and I became a star PR personality. When I received the award he was there, standing proudly next to my mom. There was such warmth in his eyes, yet it was mingled with sorrow; he suddenly seemed so small, sad, and vulnerable while my mother stood beside him, still statuesque and strong.

Barely six months later, in 1964, my father suffered a more serious stroke, and our life was changed forever. No more parties with

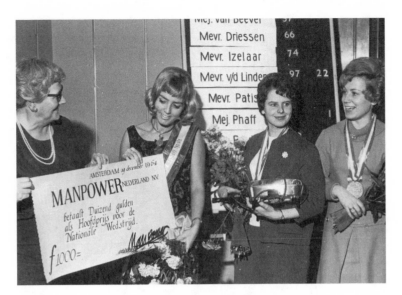

The spotlight at last

our friends or loud music in the house. Conversation dwindled to a whisper, and only quiet classical music played in the background. My father had always forecast that the day would come when he would be confined to a wheelchair as a consequence of a stroke. Now his fears were coming true.

Eight years later a journalist visiting his own mother in the hospital noticed in the same ward the tiny, paralyzed man who was my father. By now he had suffered his fifth stroke, but when the journalist discovered his identity, he persuaded my mother to give him an interview. The poignant story of the transformation of this once-prominent psychiatrist into the helpless patient became the subject of a full-page article in one of the country's most respected newspapers. This brought my father's condition to the attention of thousands of readers who had been his patients, or knew of him by reputation—and the most generous among them took up a collection that grew large enough at last to buy my mother an automobile built to accommodate the wheelchair that carried my father.

16

My Ordeal

(Mick's Narrative)

A doctor can soothe the anxieties of a patient with reassuring words; the one person to whom he can give no hope, provide no comfort, is himself. I had felt my strength ebbing, my old pains growing more persistent, and facing each day was a more demanding ordeal. I knew I could not go on but hoped I might cheat fate for at least a few years by moving the family to Valencia, where the glowing warmth of the sun might bring some relief to my aching body.

Then came the first of my strokes. Even a mild stroke is a traumatic experience, for sufferer and family alike, but I could manage the slight paralysis and was assured that I could look forward to a complete recovery. Still, as a doctor I suspected what old age might hold in store for me, so I decided to abandon our Spanish idyll and get back to Amsterdam as quickly as possible. I told Germaine I wanted to return to support Xaviera during the Manpower competition, but in truth I was also anxious to move back to Holland: Dutch hospitals and medical care were superior to what was available in Spain, and I felt sure that sooner or later I would require careful attention.

Still, my health was not yet so impaired that I couldn't get around, and I was standing there beside Germaine in the crowded hall as the judges selected Holland's best secretary. There was a hush of excitement; knowing how hard she had worked to reach the finals, of course, I was nursing every hope that my daughter would win. I needn't have worried: Xaviera possessed a dogged determination to succeed, and this competition had certainly sparked off all her competitiveness. When her triumph was announced and she stepped up to collect her prize in front of the assembled press and TV cameras, my eyes were filled with pride and tears. But what touched me more deeply than I can describe were her words whispered in my ear as she came over, still clutching the check: "I did it for you, Pappi."

I THINK WE ALL REGRETTED not being able to move back into our old house on the Nassaukade, though we were fortunate that my former colleague's widow offered us her place just when we were desperately seeking a new home. Still, the Slotermeer is a working-class district, with none of the charm of the neighborhood where we had lived and worked for all those years since our return from Indonesia. Like Xaviera, Germaine also had great willpower, and it was her determination that turned this dull, unattractive dwelling into something special. She reclaimed our furniture and possessions—including all my books and even my paintings—and being surrounded by them once more brought me both comfort and security.

Xaviera was less contented. Her bedroom was partitioned off from the main dining area by a heavy purple curtain, but she resented not being able to shut her door and retreat into her own private world. Not that she ever enjoyed complete privacy anyway, since Germaine always had the key to her room, enabling her to keep a watchful eye on our daughter's escapades—real or imagined. But we all three settled down, determined to make the best of it.

I knew I had to take things easy, to moderate the pace of life I had

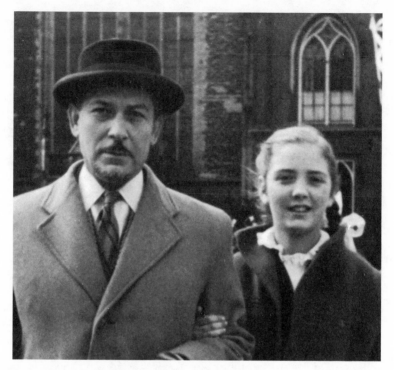

Strolling the streets with Mick

enjoyed as a young man. My blood pressure remained persistently high, and Xaviera, young as she was, worried at the sight of the veins standing out on my forehead. The massages she gave me expressed her love through the tips of her fingers, but the relief soon passed.

I feared the worst, and it wasn't long before the blow fell. Sudden stabbing pain, blackness, then nothing. I have no recollection of how long I was unconscious. I heard voices—strange men who seemed to be hovering over me. At first there was just noise and confusion; then I began to make out intelligible words, something about getting no reaction, and I realized they were talking about me. I wanted to open my eyes, but there was some kind of pressure on them—or was I too weak even to lift my eyelids? I gathered what strength I had, and with one despairing effort forced them to flutter open for an instant. There were two men bending over me, one shining a flashlight into my eyes. I tried to turn away but could not stir a muscle. My limbs were numb. And then I knew.

This stroke was very different. The whole of the left side of my body was paralyzed, though I could see and hear what was going on around me. I was lying on a couch; I must have been in a room upstairs, since I could hear Germaine's voice calling down to Xaviera. Then my wife and my daughter were at my side weeping; there was fear in their eyes, yet I could utter not a word to reassure them. Pain racked my body, but it was the sense of complete helplessness that devastated my mind. I had lived such an active life; was I to end my days as a living mummy, cut off from my family and friends? Or worse, would my reason—my very consciousness—disintegrate, leaving me no better than a vegetable?

Germaine and Xaviera were so happy I hadn't died that the full realization of what lay ahead took time to dawn on them. But it wasn't long before they fully shared my anguish. The chatter and hubbub of family life gave way to subdued whispers; where there had been happy music, now silence reigned. The curtains were drawn, as if my room were already a death chamber. Instead of the companionship of a meal around the table, I had to endure the indignity of being spoon-fed.

After a time I regained some minimal control over my right hand; I could speak, though my voice was little more than a whisper, and my mind was quite clear. This life could not continue; my condition was such that I required constant skilled medical attention. So when the ambulance arrived to take me to the hospital in Hilversum, where there were specialists and facilities to tend me, I made my decision. The stroke had shattered the illusions I had cherished. Good God, hadn't I been a doctor for all those years? I knew that surviving this stroke only meant I would have to suffer another, and then another, each carving away another shred of hope. My one concern now was to shield Germaine and Xaviera from the pain and stress of watching the inexorable decay of my body—and, most likely, the eventual clouding of my mind. Better to end it, I thought, while I still retained some dignity and the freedom to choose.

But how? I hadn't the strength to clamber out of bed, let alone the agility to hang myself. There was no open razor at hand, and even if I had one I couldn't have managed to handle it. I certainly couldn't appeal to Xaviera or Germaine to be my accomplice. Whatever I would use had to be within reach, on my bedside table, something I could pick up and hide before being lifted onto the stretcher and carried to the ambulance.

HAVING RESOLVED to end my life, I now confronted the grim irony of being dispatched to a rehabilitation center. And in my deep despair, could they have chosen a place with a more wildly inappropriate name than Zonnestraal: Sunbeams!

I had always been an active person, even nervous, unaccustomed to keeping still for long periods except when actively meditating. But now I needed patience. The long hours cooped up in the bare room, staring in silence at blank white walls, seemed a preview of death itself, and the emptiness of this life only sharpened my determination to act as soon as possible. My chosen instrument was a bedside alarm clock, which I'd smuggled into this drab house of sunbeams. It was hardly likely to rouse suspicions if it should be discovered by a nurse; all I had to do was find a moment when I could be alone and undisturbed—and with the hospital's chronic staff shortage, that posed little problem.

I waited until I had recovered enough strength to pull myself into a sitting position; my left side was still completely paralyzed, but I used my right hand to grasp a bar suspended over the bed and lift myself up. In my weakened state, it took several days before I was able to struggle up and release the bar without slipping back in the bed—and to smash the glass of the clock against the iron bed frame. Several splinters of glass had fallen onto the floor, but I managed to hold on to a few jagged fragments sharp enough to sever an artery. I was so weak from my exertions that I had to rest for what seemed ages before I could summon up the mental and physical strength to make that final decisive stroke.

The monotony of my confinement was broken by visits from

Germaine and Xaviera, who made the forty-five-minute journey from Amsterdam every other day, and I waited until a day when I knew they weren't coming. Then, with my one sound hand, I hacked at my throat. It was a messy business. I didn't have enough control to make a good clean cut: I'd been expecting a torrent of blood, but all I managed was a trickle that seeped onto the sheet and smeared my neck and shoulders. Still, I was convinced the wounds were deep enough to take my life, and I sobbed with anguish and yet with relief that my courage hadn't failed me.

Suddenly the door opened, and Xaviera walked in. My first reaction was to pull the sheet up in a futile attempt to hide the bloodstains, but the anxiety in my eyes was enough to alert her that something was dreadfully wrong. Running over to the bed, she pulled the sheet down and gazed in horror.

"Oh my God, Pappi, what have you done to yourself!"

She noticed the pieces of glass on the floor, and looked at the bedside table. "Where is the alarm clock?" she demanded. Then she put it all together. "You mean you actually tried to kill yourself with that?"

One glance at my face told her the whole sorry story. I'd never known such grief. My only intention was to spare my loved ones any distress, and all I had managed was to inflict suffering upon my daughter.

"What made you come today, of all days?" I said, sobbing.

"I had a premonition that something dreadful was about to happen," she said. "You know that even when you're not with us, I know what's going on in your mind. I knew it, Pappi, I just knew it. That's why I nagged Mom to drive over today rather than wait until tomorrow. Why did you do it, Pappi?" she asked.

"Haven't I caused you and your mother enough tsuris?" The Yiddish word seemed so much more expressive than *sorrow*. "Don't you understand? All that's left for me to look forward to is one stroke after another, until the last one kills me. And every time I become more of a burden. I went to Valencia to live; I had to come back to Holland to die."

My voice was so weak that she had to lean over to hear my words. If Germaine had walked in and seen me in that state, she would have broken down in hysterics, so Xaviera tenderly wiped the blood from my face with a damp cloth and stroked my hair.

"We know you've had your naughty moments, Daddy, and we've had our share of troubles. But you must know we love you. We would miss you so much. Please promise you'll never do anything so foolish again."

How could I deny her? Of course I wanted to go on living with my wife and daughter, and I knew I was too weak to steel myself for another attempt. I nodded; Xaviera smiled encouragement and kissed me. Then she called for assistance. Nurses were summoned, and my wounds dressed; a doctor pronounced my condition serious but not fatal. Criminals are often condemned to die; I was condemned to live.

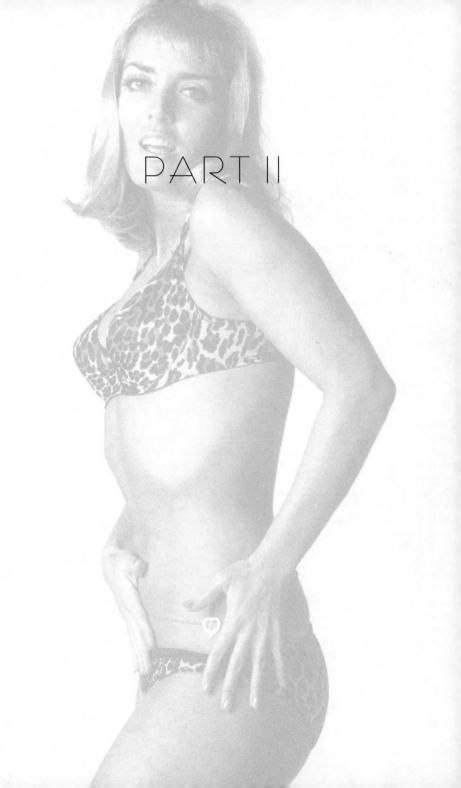

PART II

17

Mother and Daughter

THROUGHOUT my childhood, it was my father I idolized. He so dominated my emotions that I resented even my mother's presence as an intrusion on our intimacy. Yet in the days of my father's illness there grew up a bond between us so strong that we seemed to share each other's thoughts and pains even when we were at opposite ends of the earth.

When Mick suffered the first of his strokes, Germaine rose valiantly to the challenge of becoming the strong partner. I was just twenty, and couldn't face the sight of his gradual disintegration. I took refuge in adventures with boyfriends.

By then, too, I had discovered my bisexuality. In truth, the seeds were planted in high school; math and science held no thrill for me, but I came to life in art classes, where I responded to my teacher Betty. Betty was the first woman I knew to wear a khaki pantsuit; the only women who wore pants in those days were celebrities like Marlene Dietrich or Greta Garbo, who were notoriously bisexual. Betty pretended to be engaged to one of Holland's most famous opera singers; later he turned out to be quite gay himself, but being engaged to him freed her to pursue a lesbian lifestyle without fear of stigma. After I'd left school Betty and I chanced to meet on a beach at Zandvoort, and she became my first female lover.

So now that I'd grown up, there were diversions aplenty—if I could make the time to find them. My mother, of course, had grown preoccupied with caring for her husband, liberating me from her stifling watchfulness. But now I hankered for a fuller life, away from the confines of Holland. Amsterdam was no backwoods village, but it hadn't yet become a swinger's paradise. In short, I was bored.

Twelve years after the end of the war, my stepsister Mona—Mick's daughter from his first marriage—had tracked him down through the Red Cross and came from South Africa with her new husband to visit her long-lost father. Their reunion was highly emotional, and as they embraced, Germaine was gnawed by pangs of jealousy. I had similar feelings, of course, but retaliated by flirting outrageously with Jon, Mona's handsome husband—which only annoyed Germaine more.

My father's declining health marked a real crisis in my life. Whatever social or sexual conquests or defeats I encountered outside, my life at home—with our weekend outings to Café Eylders, and the comfort of our everyday routine—had been the rock on which I relied, and I had learned to live with my parents' occasional quarrels. But I was absolutely unprepared for anything so devastating as Mick's stroke. I feared that his breakdown might undermine the very foundations of our life as a family. And so, bored with Amsterdam and panicked by my home life, I felt compelled to escape.

I'd recently been talking with some friends who'd just returned from South Africa, enraptured by the sunshine and beaches. So when I learned that the South African government would pay airfare for would-be immigrants, I decided the time had come to fly the coop and get the hell out of Holland.

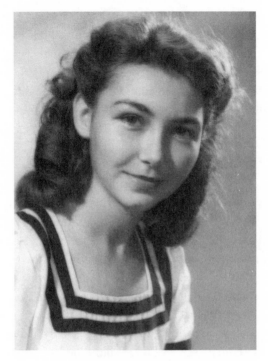

My half sister Mona

Mona and I had taken an immediate liking to each other—despite my flirting with her husband—so when I proposed coming to Johannesburg to stay with the couple and their three children, I was given a warm welcome. I've always been a sun worshipper, and basking by the pool was a joyful relief from the long, dark days of the Dutch winter. The outdoor life in South Africa delighted me, and I sought distraction in every kind of physical activity: swimming, walking, and cycling, dancing and socializing. I even had my Heinkel motor scooter, zippy enough to satisfy my passion for speed, shipped down from Holland.

I suppose that ever since my romp in the haystack with Rudolf, I had found relief from tension or depression in sex. I may have been a late starter, but now I was making up for lost time—and

there was no shortage of willing and able partners in Johannesburg.
I grew concerned that Mona might suspect me of having designs on
her husband—and, after all, a nubile twenty-one-year-old was far
more dangerous than a sexually precocious schoolgirl. So in order
to save her any anxiety I decided to find an apartment of my own—
which would, of course, free me to do whatever I pleased without
having to worry about embarrassing their sweet little family.

AT FIRST, life was fast and furious; I was having fun by night, and
working by day as an executive secretary with a large advertising
agency. When good news came from home—my father had recovered sufficiently that my mother felt able to leave his bedside and
engage a nurse to look after him—I eagerly returned for a short
visit. After months of separation I appreciated just how close a family we were, and how much I missed my mom when we were apart.
If my social life in South Africa was unfulfilling—if I was already
coming to realize how desperately I had tried to lose myself in
casual, indiscriminate sex, or how disillusioned I had become with
men who were incapable of anything more than hopping into bed
with any woman who would open her legs—I made sure my mother
had no idea of my own unhappiness.

When I returned to South Africa, I was hungry for a lasting
romance, ready to fall in love and commit myself for life to Mr.
Right. So when Carl appeared—literally tall, dark, and handsome,
an American with a well-paid, prestigious job—it was inevitable
that I'd fail to recognize him as Mr. Wrong. I fell head over heels,
and made it clear to all the beach-and-bar Romeos that I was no
longer available to them.

When Carl was asked to move to Durban for work, I went with
him, hoping to give us a chance to get to know each other more
profoundly. Looking back now, I must admit he wasn't the greatest
lover I've ever encountered, but he was well built, and so great was
our passion that I had no complaints about his initial shortcomings.

So when he proposed that I follow him back to New York—and that we get married—I was walking on air.

The trouble with walking on air is that it does let you down with a nasty bump. The truth was that Carl was entirely selfish; as I was later to discover, he was also deceitful. Sure, that first night he brought me a great bouquet of red roses—but that was before we became engaged. Once he felt he had won me, and there was no need to put himself out to please me, everything about our relationship was dictated by his convenience. We still made love, but there was less and less pretense that it was for our mutual pleasure. And when he was "too busy with business," I began to be suspicious about just what kind of business he meant.

Why, then, did I continue our affair, and make plans to join him in New York? Stressed out by my father's condition, disenchanted with so many boring South Africans who were all balls and no brains, I trusted that somehow, once we'd returned to his own country, Carl would be different and treat me with consideration and tenderness. After all, I'd promised to give up everything to follow him to a foreign country, where I had no friends and would be totally dependent on him. I had made a lifelong commitment. I simply had to believe in him.

But I could not keep my eyes shut all the time. More and more frequently, he was too much of an asshole even for me, his trusting fiancée, to put up with, and we had savage rows which reduced me to black despair. When I got too upset, I used to get away on my scooter. The thrill of driving fast, weaving through traffic, feeling the adrenaline rush of danger, gave me the kick I needed. Yet somewhere in the back of my mind there lurked the temptation to escape once and for all from unhappiness. When I was sixteen, my mother had returned from shopping to find me, purple-faced, having undertaken a half-serious, half-curious attempt to kill myself by sticking my head in the gas oven. Death—or the dying game, as I was to call it—always exercised an obsessive attraction for me, even though I enjoyed a great zest for living at the same time.

Now, blinded by pain and hopelessness, by destructive rage at Carl's latest and worst display of heartlessness and hostility, I got out and drove more wildly than ever. A big heavy truck lumbered toward me on the other side of the road. I did not consciously consider suicide, but without thinking I swung the scooter directly in its path.

The next thing I knew I was lying on the side of the road, crushed by the scooter, in a kind of dazed agony. It was a hell of a shock for the poor guy who drove the truck, and it must have been a huge relief for him when he discovered I was still alive, although I was severely concussed and had a broken leg.

Did I really want to kill myself? Did I deny that death wish at the very last moment? I don't honestly know the answer. Perhaps the will to live had won; perhaps I had unconsciously swung the handlebar at the very last moment and avoided a fatal injury. But to everyone there come moments of despair, and I know that is what was going through my head as I drove deliberately toward oblivion.

BUT I WASN'T the only member of the family to manage such a hairsbreadth escape on the road; and it was then that I first became aware of the mysterious mother-daughter union that had become part of my life.

Back in my apartment, after I had recovered, I felt a sudden stabbing pain in my chest. In my mind's eye there flashed a vision of a child knocked off her bicycle; an ambulance, siren wailing and lights flashing as it raced through the traffic, followed by my mother's car. It could not have lasted longer than a second, but it was as vivid as if I had been standing there. An hour or so later, I put in my regular call to Amsterdam to see how my dad was. My mother answered the phone. She was breathless and agitated—but, before she uttered a word, I knew what she was going to tell me.

"Xaviera, is that you?" she said.

"But she's all right, isn't she?" I demanded.

"Yes, she's badly shaken and has a few bruises," Germaine answered. Then it struck her. "But how did you know about the accident?"

I could not tell her, since I had no idea myself. But it was as clear as if I had seen her swerving and knocking the girl off her bicycle.

"She was only a kid," I said.

"Just thirteen," Germaine replied.

Learned academics may call such phenomena telepathy, or sympathy pains: I offer no explanation, merely recount what I have experienced. I could sense what had happened to my mother and what went on in her mind. Twenty years later, we would discover it could be a two-way process.

18

New York, New York!

CARL CALLED on my parents in Amsterdam and was absolutely charming. This went some way toward reassuring me after his erratic behavior in South Africa, and I began to dream again of marriage, kids, and a blissful life with the man I loved. He was waiting for me at JFK, and I pushed my way through the crowds to rush into his arms, eager for us to be reunited in one long, ecstatic kiss. Only it didn't happen that way. He seemed embarrassed, and gave me only a perfunctory peck before leading the way to his car. I was confused: Was he ashamed of me? Or was it just that people didn't embrace in public in the United States? Other couples didn't seem to have the same inhibitions. "Welcome to America," he told me, but he certainly didn't seem overjoyed to see me. There was an awkwardness, an air of reserve in his manner, that raised doubts in my mind. In the car, I asked him straight out if there was another woman. There was a long pause. Carl wasn't prepared for such a direct, no-nonsense question, but his silence alone was an admission of guilt. Then out came his story: he had slept two or three times, he said, with a woman he'd met at a conference in Jamaica. Rona was in her midthirties, and had an eight-year-old son. He didn't love her, but she was crazy about him; he had acted out of pity for her passion, though it was a love he could not return. I felt relieved that everything was out in the open—but was it?

In his penthouse we made love, but we were going through the motions. We were still lying on the bed when the phone rang, and he was more amorous toward the caller than he had been to me. After that calamitous first night, things rapidly got worse. In the morning, a Sunday, he left me alone while he went to help his mother stage an art exhibition. He never suggested that I go along. Would I have been in the way? So I waited in the apartment on my first day in the city for his promised return to take me out to dinner at six. When he returned, at ten, I was lying in bed in tears. I shouldn't have been surprised the next morning when, after he left for the office, Rona called. I introduced myself as Carl's fiancée; she explained that *she* was his fiancée. I had been clinging to the hope that Carl was slowly shaking off his past, that it would all work out, but in my heart I knew I was deluding myself. The final blow came when he took me home to meet his parents, and his mother—a confection of expensive fashionable clothes, blind prejudices, and snobbish ignorance—accused me of exploiting her son.

Exploiting *him*? I had moved in with him to wait for our wedding, and he was ready enough to go to bed with me, yet each day the wedding retreated further into the future. And Carl began to begrudge every cent, refusing even to pay for my clothes to be dry-cleaned. When my visa was about to expire, I hoped that would persuade Carl to quit procrastinating and go through with the wedding without delay. Instead he proposed that I get a job with the Dutch consulate, so that I could go on being his mistress while relieving him of the burden of supporting me financially.

In every life there come turning points, moments of decision that direct the course of one's future, and I had arrived at just such a moment. I knew I could go home to Amsterdam and carry on where I'd left off as a secretary. I had the qualifications and the experience to make a conventional career for myself and earn good money. My parents might be disappointed that I hadn't married the handsome young man they'd met, but I was sure I could count on their support once they learned the truth about this Prince Charming. I had run away after my father had suffered that severe stroke, but his condition had since stabilized, and I was starting to come to terms with the fact that he would never recover his youthful energy. Still, I couldn't help feeling that to return to my old life with my parents would be an admission of failure, an acceptance of the dim routine I had rebelled against when I took off for South Africa.

Then came the last straw: a violent showdown with Carl's mother, who hit me and threatened to have me deported. My gallant fiancé's reaction? He was furious with *me,* for "insulting" his mother.

But there was an alternative. Why go back when I could go forward? At first I'd taken umbrage at Carl's idea about getting a job, but soon I began to see it as a challenge, and I've always been ready to rise to a challenge. New York was a new world, a new life; for me, I hoped, it might be a new beginning. I got a secretarial appointment with the Dutch consulate and moved out into an apartment of my own.

As time went on, one revelation of Carl's dishonesty followed another. I learned that he wasn't legally divorced. Then, on a business trip, he had an affair with a Dutch friend I'd introduced him to and proposed marriage to her while we were still living together. His sexual behavior changed. He demanded that I abuse and assault him; he began functioning only as a masochist, which might have given him pleasure but did little for me. Earlier he'd talked of wanting us to have a child, but one day when I complained of a stomachache, he became hysterical, panicked, and threatened me, afraid that I was pregnant. I was so depressed that I took an overdose of sleeping pills. Groggily I walked to the balcony of the twenty-fifth-floor apartment, intending to leap to my death, until Carl cried out, "Don't jump! You'll make a mess all over the pavement. What will the neighbors say?"

That was enough to bring me back from the brink. Killing myself for him, I realized, would be foolish. He wasn't worth it. I'd survived the urge to commit suicide before; there was no reason to stop now.

DID THE BARRENNESS of my emotional life with Carl whet my sexual appetite? Looking back after all these years, I suppose it did. Manhattan offered plenty of opportunities for a pretty girl to indulge her libido. I had sex because I enjoyed it. And I was astonished when I discovered that you could actually make a mint by charging men in exchange for sexual pleasures. During the day I was still the ideal secretary, but no longer did I need to sit all day on what somebody once called "that gold mine."

Social life in 1960s New York was wild and fun, but it was certainly expensive, well out of reach for a young girl living on her own on a secretarial salary. So if men were ready, willing, even eager to pay me for what I wanted to do anyway, why not accept gracefully? And that, in short, was how I became the Happy Hooker.

Back home in Amsterdam, my mother had her hands full tending an invalid husband, even with her professional nursing help. I didn't want to add to her worries, and I knew from her furious reactions to my dating life in Holland that she would have gone ballistic if she had the faintest suspicion of my present nightlife. So I wrote home regularly, phoned occasionally, did all I could to set her mind at rest. If friends or neighbors asked whether she had doubts about my welfare, she had no worries: what could be more respectable than a clerical career in so staid an institution as the Dutch mission to the United Nations? To her it must have sounded as safe as a convent.

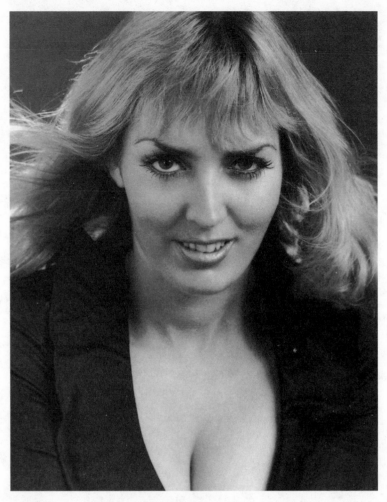

A model madam

IT DIDN'T TAKE LONG for me to discover that, whether as a hooker or as a madam, one had partners. The Mafia took their cut under threat of violence, and the police took theirs as a condition for allowing one to remain in business. Both insisted on free samples of the merchandise, and expected gratitude for the "protection" they were kind enough to provide. Being a foreigner left me particularly vulnerable: any suspicion of illegality reported to the immigration service would result in cancellation of my green card and deportation. So I needed someone to deal with these benefactors and—as I soon began to earn real money—look after my financial affairs.

The precious bond that connected me to my father, that gave me so much joy during his lifetime, also caused me much anguish while we were apart in the years of his illness. Having consigned Carl to well-earned oblivion, I missed my father more than ever—despite my self-image as an independent woman, bold enough to defy convention and to hell with the consequences. It's an ache that has returned now and again throughout my life, and at each crisis I have found consolation in the company of an older man: not so much as a substitute for my father, but as a sort of shadow of his personality, an older and wiser figure on whom I could rely. Or at least, on whom I thought I could rely at the time.

And that is how Larry entered my life. Still the very proper diplomatic secretary by day, I was now working at the Belgian mission and had earned enough to treat myself to a Christmas vacation in Puerto Rico. While I was there I happened to meet this charming, handsome man, who was making quite a splash at the gambling tables. Larry, my silver fox, was fifteen years older than me, and he knew his way around. For me Puerto Rico was a working holiday, which I enjoyed along with several of the casino's patrons. Larry and I hit it off, and the day after we met I moved into the guesthouse where he was staying.

The next day I happened to run into a shifty businessman I knew, who'd planted a phony check on me back in New York in payment for my professional services. Of course his wife was now by his side—which gave me a heaven-sent opportunity for retribution . . . and $150 in cash.

But I'd learned an important lesson: a casual client's check might not hold up any longer than his erection. From then on I worked strictly on a cash basis, and before it was time to get back to New York I'd accumulated quite a hoard of paper money. Leaving the money around was risky: three of my housemates had law degrees, but I suspected that in the face of temptation they might prove light-fingered. On the other hand there was Larry, mature, debonair, and above all, in my eyes, reliable. When we went to dinner, he paid with credit cards that were solid—although to this day I don't know for sure that they were his own.

What I do know is that I never regarded Larry as a client, or as a pimp; to me he was always my boyfriend. And so, rather than bothering to open a bank account for my short stay in Puerto Rico, I stuffed several thousand dollars in an envelope and gave it to Larry to keep safe for me.

BACK IN NEW YORK, something extraordinary happened: when I asked Larry for my money he gave it back to me, down to the last dollar. From then on he became my business manager, as well as my regular lover.

Once I had established myself as a madam in New York, I knew there could be trouble if my extramural activities should become known to the Dutch officials. Larry was there to reassure and protect me. He was an insurance adjuster, and he surely did a lot of adjusting for me. He was my intermediary with the unholy alliance of cops and crooks: when a girl got busted Larry dealt with the matter; when there was money to be invested without attracting the attention of the Internal Revenue Service, Larry placed it on the street. In short, he served as my troubleshooter—and running a bordello invariably involves trouble.

Above all, though, he was the man who took me out when I needed a break, who entertained me and helped me remain as sane as anyone can be while leading the double life of madam on the phone to clients and dutiful daughter on the phone to Mom. Things were starting to go well for me. I met a lot of influential men, often with their clothes on. There were the occasional glitches: being conveyed to the Tombs in a paddy wagon wasn't my idea of a tourist excursion, but good old dependable Larry turned up, the bail bond was paid, and my notorious black book of clients' names and particulars remained inviolate. So my life went on in the Big Apple, hectic and hyperactive as ever.

In Amsterdam, meanwhile, my father's condition had stabilized. Reassured by the reliable nursing he was receiving, my mother decided to see for herself how her daughter was faring so far from home.

When she arrived, I took every measure I could to conceal my entrepreneurial side. I took my telephone calls in a room I assured her was my office—plausible enough, since diplomatic work wasn't confined to taking notes and making appointments during office hours. This illusion of being involved with high-ranking officials explained my being able to afford a lifestyle well beyond the reach of a conventional secretary. Occasionally one of my girls dropped by, but they were always soberly dressed with discreet makeup, so they easily passed for normal social acquaintances. Germaine may have thought I'd made rather a lot of friends, but New York is a friendly city, and she knew I was a friendly person.

Initially, Larry made a great impression on her. He was a smooth operator and knew how to exploit his charm. As a treat, he took both of us for a weekend to Las Vegas. After the troubles she had endured, the bustle of the place with its teeming casinos gave Germaine a break she badly needed. Larry was in his element at the tables, and Germaine joined in the frenzied spirit. She was too cautious to have the true gambling temperament, but she abandoned her usual reserve enough to try her luck with the slot machines, and soon graduated to roulette. While Larry was instructing me in blackjack, she was doing very nicely at the wheel. When we rejoined her she was sitting behind a substantial mound of chips, a glint in her eye.

Now it was I who had to counsel caution. "Quit while you're

ahead, Mama—you know what they say about beginner's luck."
She was reluctant but, with some regrets, yielded to a bit of hard-
headed Dutch prudence. She shook her head at the croupier, gathered up her chips, and cashed them in. In her heart she knew I'd
certainly saved her from giving back all her winnings and perhaps
more, so she used her windfall to buy a beautiful watch as a present for me.

Back in New York Larry took us out to a lavish dinner at the
Waldorf-Astoria. The food was excellent, and the service matched
the lavish tip Larry produced with a flourish. We had a choice table
and were treated royally by everybody from the maître d' down to
the humblest waiter. I admired Larry's flamboyance, grateful to see
him putting on such a show for my mother.

Back home, though, I learned she didn't share my enthusiasm.

"What do you mean, he was generous?" she asked.

For once, I was really annoyed by my mother's attitude. How
could she fail to appreciate Larry, when he'd pulled out all the stops
to show us such a good time? Could she be jealous? After all, Larry
was nearer her age than mine.

She shook her head in bewilderment. "You mean you didn't tell
him to take that money from your safe? He had the key, so I
thought you must have arranged it with him."

I'd had a little safe built into the wall beside my bed and had
given Larry a key so that he could deposit cash there when I was
busy. Germaine had been inside my walk-in closet choosing something to wear, she said, when Larry stole into the bedroom, went to
the safe, and took out a fistful of hundred-dollar bills.

"He never saw me," she explained. "And since he had the key,
who was I to ask questions?"

I couldn't see how Germaine could have been mistaken, yet I
didn't want to believe her. Telling myself this was all the product
of her suspicious mind and negative attitude, I condemned her
for spying on my boyfriend. I'd built up such trust in Larry that I

made myself believe there must be some innocent explanation. But I didn't confront him—that could have shattered my illusions, and I wasn't prepared for that.

From then on I watched my money more carefully, though, and eventually I had to face the reality of Larry's thieving ways. Still, I couldn't bring myself to condemn *him*. Sure, he lived on his wits and stole from my petty cash; but he enlivened my life, and he was loyal to me in his fashion. Besides, I had a lot more money than he did, and since his pilfering was modest, I could afford to turn a blind eye. After all, Larry did have a generous disposition; it's just a shame he was generous with my money, not his own.

19

Watergate Watershed

IF I LEARNED anything beneficial during my time with Carl, it was that for a woman offering fantasy sex, pain plus pleasure equals profit. And I must admit that I began to find sadomasochism a turn-on—as long as I literally held the whip hand. Being abused and humiliated could produce the height of ecstasy for Carl, though I wonder if he ever asked himself, "What would the neighbors think?"

Germaine was soon to find out, with a jolt, just what *her* neighbors thought. Now that Mick's adventurous life was a thing of the past, her days passed quietly and uneventfully. That is, until one day a kind friend brought to her notice a story in *De Telegraaf,* a widely read Dutch daily that specializes in ferreting out stories about the private lives of celebrities. And there, of all things, was a photograph of her daughter in her working clothes—not the demure costume of the sober secretary, but full war paint, black leather boots, sexy underwear ... and brandishing a vicious-looking whip. It was a great story, at least for the journalist: "Our

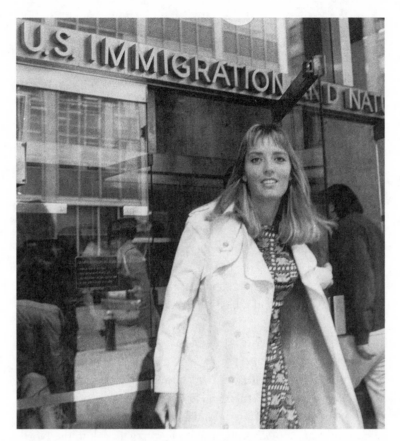

Leaving the immigration building

own Vera de Vries," it cried, was none other than the notorious Xaviera Hollander, author of the internationally scandalous memoir *The Happy Hooker*. I can't honestly say I know what my mother's reactions were in that moment—I was a thousand miles away at the time—though before too long she seemed somehow to reconcile herself to my lifestyle and newfound notoriety. But I'm sure Germaine must have appreciated the thoughtfulness of such good neighbors.

It was just as the Watergate scandal was at its peak in 1972 that

The Happy Hooker, a book I had decided to write about my experiences in New York, filled the bookshops and hit the headlines. The pure and the prurient licked their lips in anticipation: with the televised hearings whetting their appetites for the secrets of the rich and powerful, I'm sure they were eager to hear me reveal the names of public figures who'd paid me or my girls for sex. They were disappointed. As far as I was concerned, what went on in my house was my affair; my business was private and confidential, and despite enormous pressure I refused to name names and join in the witch-hunt. And so I became one of the hunted and was hounded out of the country.

I stayed briefly in London with Bob Guccione, where I took a starring role in the Play Girl scenes he hosted in his new Penthouse Clubs. Soon he offered me the post of sexual adviser to *Penthouse,* the magazine he'd recently launched, and I've continued to write its monthly advice column, "Call Me Madam," to this day without a break.

Much has been written about swinging London, but I was accustomed to the frantic pace of New York, and London life seemed drab by comparison. And I found the casual, superficial acquaintances I made there no substitute for the warmth and friendliness of my old crowd. So when I was invited to do a highly rated Canadian TV talk show, I was eager to get back to the North American scene.

SHORTLY after my arrival, I was a guest at one of those after-hours parties where TV personalities shone in their most glamorous outfits, and I was duly dressed to kill. To be honest, I found most of the guests pretty phony; but there was one young man I met there—Paul was his name—who felt the same way; he seemed awkward in the crowd and made his escape as soon as he could.

I learned that Paul owned an antiques shop, so a few days later I sauntered over to his shop and looked in. His relief at seeing me without any makeup, hair in pigtails and feet in sandals, was palpable. We fell in love on the spot. Nine years my senior, he too reminded me of my father; though he couldn't match Mick's vivacity or breadth of knowledge, I was attracted by his honesty and independence of character. As I got to know him better, I realized that Paul was a stubborn, staid bachelor, and maybe that very challenge was what made me determined to marry him.

In stark contrast to my father, Paul was largely self-educated; he would painstakingly read "difficult" texts, consult dictionaries, analyze, absorb unfamiliar words, and incorporate them into his own vocabulary. Even writing a letter involved using a thesaurus, so it was hardly surprising when the finished product—the product of hours of labor—sometimes lacked spontaneity. He shunned the limelight in which I unashamedly reveled, so I was deprived of the pleasure of taking him to the glamorous events to which I was constantly invited. He refused to accept the role of Mr. Hollander and lived in wonder that the woman he eventually married could flip so effortlessly from Vera Jekyll to Xaviera Hyde. For him I was a private person: simple, fun-loving Vera de Vries.

My routine never varied: after my customary afternoon nap, followed by a hot bath and the ritual of putting on my makeup, I would emerge as La Hollander, ready and eager to paint the town red. I was staying in the Carriage House Hotel, a melting pot of colorful, often noisy gay boys. Soon after I moved in, the boys started looking to me for comfort and relationship advice, and the press started calling me the Bette Midler of Toronto. I was even elected to the jury for the annual Travesty Ball, which was held in the discotheque of the hotel.

At such occasions I was escorted not by Paul, who was far too conservative and straight, but by Georgie Porgy, my dazzlingly extroverted gay Hungarian photographer friend, who exhibited huge photo blowups of me in the window of his Yonge Street studio. We were self-styled raving queens, icons of the gay scene. When I was called on to officiate as judge at drag-queen parties, the kids would come to weep on my shoulder for consolation—not the sort of conduct likely to woo Paul. But I always returned to him, and he seemed to accept that beneath my glitzy persona there was a real person who loved him.

Eventually, though, Paul asked that I make up my mind: sex queen or faithful wife. I knew what I wanted, so I moved out of the hotel to join him in a luxurious penthouse apartment. But I agreed to help keep the press in the dark about our marriage; his parents were very Orthodox Jews, and Paul assured me that if his mother were to learn the news she would suffer an immediate and fatal heart attack.

AFTER MY disastrous interlude with Carl, and the exposure of Larry's light fingers, Germaine naturally wanted to check out my latest partner—especially since he was the first man to whom I'd made the commitment of marriage. Leaving her faithful friend and cleaning lady Greet in charge of the house, she came to Toronto for a visit. No doubt relieved at Paul's quiet, unassuming character, she took to him at once, and I was pleased by the friendly consideration he showed her.

To show my mom something of the glorious Canadian countryside in May, Paul drove us out on trips to the lakes. One weekend he took us to a place called Collingwood, not far out of town, where we joined some friends tapping maple trees for syrup. After a while my mother and I left them and returned to laze in the sun; I relaxed in a hammock and we drank in the tranquillity of the place. Germaine loved me to do her nails, so I climbed down to join her. Her skin glowed from the warmth of the sun, and I bent over to drink in the musky fragrance of her body. I played with her hair, trying to pin it up the way I remembered it from childhood.

Then it was my turn to be pampered. My mother gently rubbed oil on my hands to make them smooth and soft; then I lay down with my head on a cushion and my feet in her lap, and she massaged them with the soothing, sweet-smelling ointment. During such precious moments my mom and I grew ever fonder of each other. We loved to talk for hours about the past in Holland and Indonesia, about my dad in the days when he enjoyed good health. I would close my eyes and listen to Germaine retelling stories we'd both lived through, memories so vivid it was as if a film were flashing through my mind. She was a wonderful storyteller: her voice was soft and soothing, and if she forgot some detail I would take over and fill it in for her. We perfectly complemented each other, like a couple of kids who had to be close to each other.

Only when she started to become sentimental did I grow edgy. "Oh, Veraatje!" she sighed. "If you only knew how much I love you. You are all I really live for. How I love being here and having you to myself, undisturbed by other people. You've always been so restless. Even as a child I could never get you to sit still for a minute. When I wanted to reach out to you, you were like water running through my fingers. No one could ever hold you down; you always seemed to be running after something—God knows what! And yet today in the country you seem so relaxed, so peaceful."

"You'd prefer that we be shackled together, confined away from everybody, left to our own devices?" I challenged.

"Something like that," she answered dreamily. "If only Mick could be with us here, drinking in the beauty of this place."

As if to snap us out of our reverie, a few days later—in the middle of May—it actually snowed. We had been bathed in bright sunlight, gazing up at a lush green canopy of trees, when suddenly it clouded over and a soft blanket of dazzling white snow started to fall, covering everything. We held hands, amazed at the beauty of the scene and the sense of vast empty space. It was majestic and silent, as if the trees had been magically transformed into the pillars of an immense natural cathedral.

Then, just as suddenly, the sun broke through again, and all around there was a strange, gentle hissing sound. I looked up and realized that what I was seeing and hearing was the snow beginning to melt. Scattered on the damp earth lay dead wasps and bees that had been caught by the freak snowfall. I was so inspired by the magic of the singing snow that I wrote a poem to celebrate: "I Could Hear the Snow Melt."

Back in the city, though, my own storm clouds were beginning to gather.

20

Two Deaths

MY FATHER kept his promise never again to attempt to take his own life, but now there was little danger: whatever his anguish may have been, he was no longer physically capable of effective action. His friend Simon Vestdijk had a horror of hospitals, but his creative life had been so intimately linked to Mick that now he was compelled to visit his bedside. He asked Germaine to be allowed to be left alone with Mick, and they were together for half an hour. Nobody knows whether he was able to communicate with his stricken friend, but when he emerged Germaine could see how shaken he had been by the encounter. He did not need to speak; his tear-stained face said everything. The only other visitor was Uncle Julius, but Mick was too far gone to be able to respond even to him.

Mick's doctors could do nothing to restore their patient's health, and rather than keeping him confined in the impersonal hospital, they released him to his home and his wife, to be surrounded by his paintings, his books, and all the familiar objects that had been so dear to him. At first nurses came to attend him, but a fifth stroke had left him speechless, immobile, and incontinent; even his teeth had been removed. It was clear that during his last days he would best be served by loving care rather than medical expertise. So the burden of tending to the needs of this mute, motionless human wreck fell on the shoulders of Germaine, supported by Greet. It must have been the most terrible period of my mother's life, watching as her man wasted away. In the prison camp there had always been hope that the terror would pass; now there was nothing to look forward to but the ultimate liberation of death. Vestdijk came one more time, but now he too was failing, and shortly after the visit Germaine learned of his death.

Their ordeal forged a very close bond between Germaine and Greet, but this comradeship proved to have its dark side. Ever since their days in Indonesia, when Mick had jokingly suggested that Germaine was a trifle too fond of drink, she had been careful never to have more than an occasional glass of wine or medium sherry. I had seen her cheerful after a drink, but never drunk. Greet, on the other hand, was a gin-and-tonic woman, and she persuaded Germaine to join her in escaping from her misery into an alcoholic haze. So instead of one or two glasses of sherry during the day, Germaine slipped into the habit of a regular series of gin and tonics. The two of them would smoke incessantly as they were getting tipsy, but all Germaine achieved was to put on weight and suffer fits of melancholy. Fortunately the trained nurses were still in attendance, for there were times when both women were too befuddled to be of any use when help was needed. Greet's husband saw what was happening and read her the riot act, but to no avail.

One night, when the others had gone, Germaine staggered off to bed and tripped over the basket in which our dog—named Trippie, aptly enough—was sleeping. As she fell she smashed her head against the metal bar of Mick's hospital bed. The look of reproach in his eyes as he was startled awake, and no doubt smelled the alcohol on her breath, finally brought her to her senses. Germaine had cut her upper lip, but she was sufficiently sobered by the shock to phone Greet and ask her to take her to the hospital, where her wound was stitched. The scar remained with her until the day she died, as if to remind her of the mad moment of irresponsibility brought about by her sorrow. That was the end of her heavy drinking, and Greet was so stunned that she followed suit.

NEWLY REFORMED, Germaine and Greet were soon out and about during the day, shopping, paying a visit to the hairdresser, now and then calling on Julius, who had recently lost his beloved Indonesian wife and was grateful for the company. But this relief did not last long. A final massive stroke, the sixth, left Mick totally paralyzed and too weak to be moved back into hospital.

From then until the end, Greet stayed the night. Germaine dismissed the nurses, and the two women kept an eternal vigil by the sickbed. All night Greet sat up, alert for any sign of movement from Mick, while during the day Germaine would try patiently to spoon baby food between his lips to sustain the faint spark of life that remained.

His condition grew worse until at last the doctor, a family friend for more than twenty years, knew the time had come. Germaine was in tears, clutching his almost lifeless body as a mother would her drowning child.

"Germaine," he said softly, "please stop trying to feed Mick."

"Why? He is mine, isn't he?" retorted the distraught woman. "So I can do what I want with him. He has managed to eat until now, little as it was, but he is still alive, isn't he?" Her tone became shrill and aggressive. "Tell me then one good reason why I should stop feeding him."

"Germaine," he said, sighing, "have a good look at him. That is not a human being anymore. He is ninety-nine percent clinically dead. Please, let him go. What you are doing is simply torture—for him, for yourself, even for me. Can't you see? Mick cannot go on living, and he doesn't want to."

He took Mick's hand—now no more than a tiny claw—in his own and gazed down at the shriveled body. Mick was barely breathing; his features were skeletal; his Indonesian tan now a deathly pallor. His eyes remained closed, sunk in their hollow sockets; his nose seemed to have grown larger and more prominent.

"No!" Germaine screamed hysterically.

Greet took her by the shoulders, walked her over to her bed next to Mick's, and almost forced her to lie down. Germaine's voice became no more than a subdued splutter.

"I won't let go of him. I *won't* let go of him. At last he's now all mine. No one in the world wants him anymore. They can't take him away from me. He has become my baby."

The doctor went to where she lay sobbing uncontrollably. He took a hypodermic syringe from his case and gave her an injection. She quickly grew calmer and then fell into a tranquil sleep. When she woke up an hour later, Mick had peacefully died.

I HAD MADE several trips to Holland to be with my father, but the end came so suddenly that I had no opportunity to fly home. I was on a lecture tour in Edmonton, resting in my room before meeting an audience, when my mother phoned with the news. I had no time to grieve: I had hardly replaced the receiver when I was called to go and deliver the lecture. Somehow I got through with my speech, but then came the questions.

"What did your parents think when they learned you'd become a hooker?" one outraged citizen demanded.

"A few minutes before coming onto this platform, I learned that my father had died," I answered. "Maybe this is not the best time to answer that sort of question."

I don't think the audience was aware of the effort I was making to hold back my tears, but I was relieved that the questions ceased and I was able to get back to my room and my grief. There I wrote my father a letter of farewell, as much for my own sake as for his. Using a pet name for my father, Pipadoxi—it was the name of a

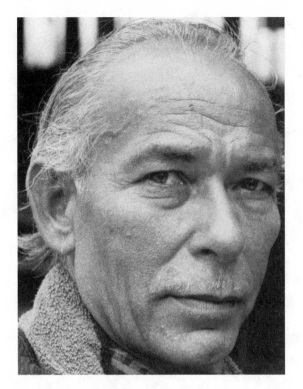

Mick in Valencia

patent medicine he once used, but I liked the sound of it—I found a piece of paper and began to write.

Dear Pipadoxi,

Across an ocean, in a country unfamiliar to you, I'm struggling to accept the truth that at last you're at peace forever. I can't control my tears; my heart literally aches; and somehow I feel closer than ever to you, you whom I've loved so much.

In a harsh, anonymous hotel room, with nothing to remind me of you or of home—not even the menorah you gave me so long ago to carry as a reminder of our Jewish ancestry. I was having bad dreams, a nightmare, intuitively I felt it coming—and then the phone call.

"My child, it's happened," Mama said calmly. "Your father died this afternoon at four. He won't suffer anymore, poor soul."

For a moment I froze; then the tears came.

"Please don't cry, Xaviera . . . talk to me!" begged Mama.

I asked how it happened. Just flesh and bones she said you were, with one attack after another. Then for twenty-four hours she never left you, till you finally slipped away. We all knew it was about to happen, of course, but the truth was so hard to accept.

And so, across the thousands of miles of telephone cable, we tried to comfort each other, until finally in grief and exhaustion we whispered good-bye.

When I was ten, I started calling you Pipadoxi. And you were always the man I admired, adored, and envied. Your wit, intelligence, charm, and warmth have always been my inspiration. You were a devoted husband, a bon vivant, a bohemian in your own way. Your many patients, for whom you worked endlessly and selflessly, stand as monuments to your skill as a physician by their own good health. And I remember the crazy times: late at night, you and Mama dancing; you without your reading glasses, playing the piano and missing the odd key. There were the rough spots too, as in every marriage, but they never lasted long. You were the first man I ever saw weeping.

Look, it's me crying now—tears of rage, sorrow, frustration, and relief. You, who did so much to ease the suffering of others, you suffered longest and most yourself. Poor Mama, too; she never wavered in her love for you, and devoted every moment of her life to caring for you these past years. What justice is there? You suffered so much in the camp during the war, surely that was enough for a lifetime!

But I remember you happy, playing with Trippie along the beach. Or with me, hand in hand during our summer holidays, teaching me new languages ... or impulsively embracing and hugging Mama in the street. And I remember you at work, rushing out of the house in any weather to heal the sick and comfort the infirm.

Then your first stroke, and suddenly it was you who were sick and infirm. And, dear Pipadoxi, how you suffered these past eight years! Unable to face it, I couldn't stay in Amsterdam, and I left Mama alone to care for you. Can you ever forgive me? Dear Papa, farewell. My love for you will never grow less. Wherever your spirit is now, watch over me with affection, please. I still desperately need your love and understanding and approval.

Your depressed, lonely, loving daughter,
Your Xaviera

For the next two years, I tried to put my life back together. No one could ever replace my Pipadoxi, but I had a husband and our own home, and I began to dream about becoming a loving parent. And then, just maybe, my child would love me as I had loved my father. But the powers that be had other ideas.

Adopting a lifestyle of domestic bliss did not save me from official persecution. Just as the Americans had got rid of me, there was pressure on the Canadian authorities to follow suit. Returning from a trip to Mexico, I was interrogated by an immigration officer, who produced a copy of *The Happy Hooker*.

"Did you write this book?" he asked.

"Sure, of course I did." I had never made a secret of my authorship.

"Claims to be your memoirs. So all those things you wrote about—did they actually happen?"

"Yes. That's why the book became something of a sensation," I replied with due modesty.

An older and wiser woman, I know now that indulging in casual conversation with inquisitive officials can be dangerous. Admitting that the contents of the book were fact, not fiction, was enough to give the Canadian government an excuse to proclaim me a self-confessed "criminal," subject to deportation as an undesirable alien. If they accepted that my sexploits were facts, I protested, it was absurd to pretend I was *undesirable*—but unfortunately they lacked a sense of humor.

I didn't find the situation all that amusing either. Once again I was hounded and denounced; my life fell again under the scrutiny of the self-righteous and evil-minded. I needed support, and my husband rose to the occasion, shielding me as well as he could from the consequences of my honesty while trying to deal with the legal consequences. In vain I protested that I'd never committed any misdemeanor in Canada, and all I wanted was the right to settle down in peace with my husband, raise a family, and continue my career as a writer. And having a child was what I desired just then, more than anything else in the world.

When I told Paul how desperately I wanted to have a baby, at first he refused to discuss the matter. I felt a growing tension between us; looking back I suppose it was inevitable, in light of our vastly different lifestyles and family backgrounds. His parents and grandparents were Polish Jewish refugees, with a strict conservative outlook, and Paul shared their appetite for a quiet way of life and simple pleasures. Often we visited friends of his who lived way out in the country and subsisted in primitive farmhouses, often without hot water. Their way of life might have been picturesque, but with just one old-fashioned stove in the kitchen, the bedrooms were freezing cold in the winter, and during the summer they got hot and steamy and were infested by millions of mosquitoes.

I had always been a city girl, fond of a city's hectic pace and exotic characters. I wanted to share all this with Paul, but when we went out for a meal he insisted on going Dutch, even though he knew my taste ran to restaurants far beyond the means of a struggling antiques dealer. It was an enormous contrast from life with Larry, who had reveled in five-star hotels, expensive restaurants, and fancy car trips, all paid for by me in hard cash. Larry was always the expansive, showy playboy; Paul was so reserved that sometimes I felt the need to demand he show me how deeply he loved me. Of course he knew all about my free sex life before we were married, and though he never complained about my affairs, eventually I realized he silently resented them, and his attitude toward me became ever more cool and cynical. It seems never to have occurred to him that his very coldness might be driving me to seek warmth in others.

At last I exploded. "Why don't you ever say 'I love you'? I need to be told. Don't you understand?"

"Xaviera, I'm still with you after all these years," he replied bitterly. "And I don't fool around. You have love affairs with girls, with boys, even the occasional older man. I never complained before we got married, but I've never gotten any pleasure from hearing about all your latest adventures—despite how often you tell me you love me! Do I need to say more?" So that was it. "Just imagine," he went on, "if we had a daughter, how would she feel when some kid at school started calling her mother the whore who wrote that dreadful book? Do you think any young girl wants that hanging over her head?"

I was struck then by the memory of what had happened, in a very similar circumstance, between my father and my mother. I was thirty-three years old; my biological alarm clock was about to ring. Like my mom, I got advice from a worldly girlfriend.

"Calculate the date of your ovulation," she told me, "then seduce him as he has never been seduced before—all night long. And stick to the good old missionary position; don't waste anything in oral sex, or way up in the air. Stick a pillow beneath you for maximum penetration, and don't rush off to rinse in the bidet afterward."

Perhaps Jane had given my mother similar advice back in Java; Germaine was far too proper to go into such intimate details. Just like her, though, I knew absolutely after Paul's ejaculation that night that I was pregnant.

My father, once he had recovered from the shock, had rejoiced in his impending paternity. But my husband, Paul, leaped with horror, as if stung by a bee. After that tremendous climax we would indulge in many sexual variations, but he made sure never to penetrate me again.

Some women find the months when a child is ripening in their womb the emotional high point of their lives. For me it was a time of deep emotional unhappiness. Paul could never reconcile himself to the idea that I was bringing his child into the world. He felt I had tricked him, entrapped him, and his resentment grew daily. I needed loving care and warmth: all he offered was frigid indifference. Rejected by the man I loved, I turned to others for consolation; and even when I felt lonely, the thought of having a little creature all my own growing inside me comforted me and saved me from despair. Before going to sleep I would fold my hands around my belly, even though there were few visible signs that I was pregnant: I knew I was no longer alone in this world. When I was well into my third month, I bought a fabulous set of new pregnancy clothes and began sticking out my belly proudly, especially when I went out.

Finding so little affection with Paul, I looked elsewhere and found comfort in the company of Milad, an Egyptian film director and screenwriter. But his kindness could not compensate for the sterility of my life with Paul. The strain affected my health and that of my unborn child. I persevered with my pregnancy without any support from Paul—or proper medical supervision—until one evening, just after making love with Milad, I collapsed. Fainting, my body racked by agonized spasms, I was brought home to a cold reception from my husband. Leaving me with Paul, Milad told him I should be taken right away to the hospital; but I was too exhausted and happy to be home in my own bed, and Paul was too stubborn to see how ill I really was. By the time he decided the following morning to have me hospitalized, I was hemorrhaging badly, paralyzed on the entire left side of my body, and in enormous pain.

The ambulance came within fifteen minutes after his emergency call, and the doctor diagnosed it at once as a life-threatening ectopic pregnancy. In less than an hour, I was on the operating table. The crisis had been going on for nearly twelve hours; if I had waited one more hour before coming to the hospital, the doctor admonished, I would certainly have died from internal bleeding. When Paul heard that, I could hear him weep behind the screens.

The only one who was there to suffer along with me, who understood my profound misery, was my mother. As soon as she heard, she flew out to be by my side.

THE CRISIS shook Paul out of his indifference, and he genuinely realized what he had come so close to losing. But Germaine's arrival gave him the opportunity to get back to his shop and earn a living. So for a month, as I gradually fought my way back to health, I was once more my mother's child. And the bond between us once again became a lifeline, which would hold us together as long as she drew breath.

The trauma of my illness and the authorities' relentless campaign for my deportation had also put a terrible strain on Paul. He was grateful to my mother for looking after me; for her part, she showed him great kindness and consideration. Years later she would remember his taste for rollmops herring, the brand of cigarettes he smoked, just how he liked his coffee and Punt y Mes. But now he needed a break, and we saw him off for a couple of weeks to the Bahamas. The Canadian government had already ruled that I was to leave the country; in view of my condition they had charitably allowed me six weeks' grace for recuperation, but I dared not accompany my husband on his trip, quite certain that if I left the country I would never be allowed to reenter.

Ironically, had I carried my pregnancy successfully to term, the fact that I was bearing a Canadian citizen would have rendered me immune from deportation.

WHEN THE DEPORTATION ORDER was served, I was more than ready to get the hell out of the country. So, without waiting for Paul's return, my mother and I put an ad in the local newspaper announcing that Xaviera Hollander was leaving Canada for good and was selling off every last possession—from her brand-new blue Audi Fox car, her furniture and wardrobe, right down to the latest LP. Because of my high profile in Toronto I had always had an unlisted number, but now I came out into the open, and the calls poured in.

I had to keep the things that were Paul's and that I knew he liked and suited his spartan lifestyle. Everything else went, sometimes to the most unexpected people. The city's police chief had just gotten married; he snapped up my king-size bed and black silk sheets. People drove in from faraway towns, neighbors walked over, and parents brought their kids to admire the treasures—and buy copies of my book, which I cheerfully autographed for them. Paul, of course, knew nothing of this sale of the century, and I smiled to think of his amazement when he returned to find only great empty spaces in place of our well-furnished home. But his beloved oil lamp and personal furniture, such as his antique table and chair, would all be there to welcome him home, and he never watched color TV anyway.

To help, I brought in Franny, a young American girl who had become my lover and slave, and she and Germaine worked tirelessly. Germaine discovered a great talent for selling and bargaining with every sort of customer—and such was the interest in my little fire sale that the most diverse crowd showed up, all eager for a special memento. There were men who wanted some item of lingerie—my bra or panties, preferably soiled—a special commodity I didn't provide at that time—and begged me to sign them for their wives or girlfriends, using marker pens they brought themselves. There were respectable housewives, the kind who always have their hair permanently waved, who brought me baggy white boxer shorts or cotton underpants to sign *With Love* and a smudge of lipstick for their men. Bargain hunters tried to pick up albums or picture books worth seventy or eighty times what they offered; I preferred to take them back to Holland rather than feed such greed. Then there were the cadgers who, having bought something, tried to wheedle a little extra, a candleholder, a glass, anything as long as it was for free. Others wanted everything for free, bringing along big shopping baskets into which they slipped expensive garments when they thought nobody was looking. (They didn't reckon on the sharp eyes of Germaine and Franny.) Franny kept a fresh pot of coffee going for the customers and spilled a pitcher as she dived to intercept sneak-thief number six. I was carrying a pouch like a mother kangaroo, but it was stuffed with dollar bills instead of my baby.

It was only to be expected that I would receive calls from every variety of freak and fanatic, but one call had amusing consequences. He sounded like an elderly man, with a tremor in his voice.

"Do you by any chance have a few pairs of Wellington boots in your collection?"

"Yes. Do you want them?" I replied, thinking nothing of it.

"Yessss," he hissed. But then he went on, in a whisper, "But are they . . . *dirty?*"

The pair in my closet was immaculate. But my Happy Hooker experience had given me an education in how to please foot, shoe, or in this case Wellington-boot fetishists.

"Of course they are very dirty. But they'll cost you a lot of money."

"How much?" he stuttered.

"Oh, at least a hundred dollars a pair."

"As long as they have lots of mud on them."

"Of course. How many pairs do you want? You see, I've got some girlfriends."

"Oh, that will be marvelous," he said, enthused. "I can do with at least four pairs. And can I meet your friends too?"

"Maybe. But if you have friends who want furniture or regular stuff, be here the day after tomorrow at five and bring them along."

So was I still playing the Happy Hooker? Maybe, but business is business. I put the scheme to my mother and Franny. At first Germaine was reluctant to get involved in selling cheap boots at such an exorbitant price, but she was won over by my commercial flair and the farce of the situation. The following morning I sent Franny to a shoe shop around the corner to buy two pairs of boots, one pair her size, the other larger. She and Germaine put on the new boots and were ordered to tramp around the park until they were nicely caked with mud before coming home with some fresh croissants for breakfast. It was raining, and I didn't feel like going for a walk, so Franny had to go out twice more, wearing my original boots to give them the same treatment. She made the obligatory grumble, as slaves do when ordered to do something they want to do anyway, but out she went, wearing a hideous plastic raincoat. Germaine would never have submitted to such an indignity: one trudge in her Wellies was enough for her!

The old gentleman arrived, impeccably dressed, with a wicked gleam in his beady eyes. He begged Franny and me to walk around the place in our boots for about ten minutes while my mom gave him a nice cup of tea and a biscuit. He was thoroughly English, with a polished Oxford accent; I'm sure a healthy spanking would have done him a world of good. He gladly took all four pairs of boots, squeezed us gently on the cheek, and paid his four hundred dollars without a murmur. He was a sweet old man and seemed affluent enough that none of us felt a moment's guilt about taking his money. I gave my mom and Franny a hundred dollars each; they richly deserved it.

But such flashes of my old carefree self were rare during those last days in Toronto. The sadness of losing my child, and my impending banishment, were almost unbearable to me in my weak-

ened physical state. The doctor's parting words had been that I
would probably never have a child of my own. I saw now that when
my mother died, I would have no family; I would be absolutely
alone, and with me the line would come to an end. And it was
the end of my dream of a settled married life. When he returned,
Paul didn't even seem surprised at the emptiness of his own place.
We greeted each other calmly, and in a few days began divorce
proceedings. But time heals old wounds, and as we got older we
achieved a cooler relationship. When Paul visited me later in
my Spanish home, he was embraced into my circle of friends with
open arms.

Is it surprising, then, that I felt more isolated than ever, that my
nightmares returned? Once more I saw my mom behind barbed
wire; I was that lonely child again, sitting on my suitcase, crying my
heart out with no one there to hug me and wipe away my tears.
Awake I shed more tears, but at least my mother was by my side here
in Toronto, holding me close as I sobbed against her shoulder. Bitter
at my treatment by the government, I retreated to the house, avoid-
ing company like a wounded animal as I slowly recovered from my
enormous loss of blood. I was letting myself go, putting on weight,
cutting my hair so short as to completely change my appearance.

It took a few months for me to regain my self-confidence. But
back home in Amsterdam I found solace now in Betty, my old
teacher and first woman lover, who gave me the reassurance I
needed. We revived our love affair: here was someone who had
never once rejected me.

"Just because you can't have children, that doesn't mean you are
not a complete woman. Everything you've done, everything you've
written, is your own contribution to womanhood. It is every bit as
valuable as the contribution made by any mother."

I took her words to heart and started to rebuild myself physically. I began growing my hair back and worked to shed some of the
weight I had put on in the depths of my depression. One life was
over, I told myself; now I must begin another.

PART III

21

Lonely No More

AMSTELVEEN IS A SEDATE, respectable suburb of Amsterdam, worlds apart from the sex clubs and strip joints of the city center patronized by tourists, with its "brown" cafés, crowded streets, and bustling street markets. Amstelveen, with its uniformly neat houses and their well-tended gardens, is home to dentists and doctors, accountants and retired bank managers. They have an air of reasonable rather than excessive wealth. It wasn't the sort of district in which one might expect the Happy Hooker to make a home. But it suited low-profile Vera de Vries, with her cropped hair and bruised soul.

Before I could begin to build a new life, I needed a period of respite to get my act together. And the comfortable, conventional house I bought from a retired dentist helped restore the sense of security I had lost in those last days in Canada. I knew even then that this would be just a passing phase, and that before many years I would outlive my Amstelveen haven.

I turned my attention to renewing old friendships, meeting

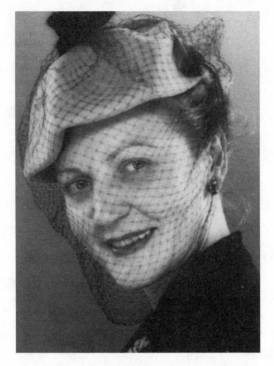

Germaine

others who had endured the Japanese occupation in Indonesia. I began to learn much of my father's ordeal, things he would never talk about himself. My mother was still reluctant to talk freely of those days. She was so relieved to have me back home, away from the constant attacks I suffered in the United States and Canada, that all she wanted was for us to enjoy the present together and look to a happier future. In our tight little family circle, my father had been the focus of our lives; no one could take his place, and in his absence we inevitably drew closer to each other. Every few days I would drive over to her house, or she would drop by to see how I was getting along, and even when we weren't together we kept the phone lines pretty busy.

We had become so close, and I knew her so well, that I could divine what was going on in her mind; often I felt I could hear her words in my head even before she said them. Yet she could still take me by surprise with her spontaneity. One occasion made such an impression on me that now, more than a year after she died, I can still close my eyes and relive the moment.

It was her birthday, and I wanted to give her something that would remind her of those love tokens from Mick she treasured so much. Both of them were heavy smokers, and although I have never touched tobacco, I had always been intrigued by the nicotine stain on my father's middle finger. He used to hold his cigarette in the Indonesian manner, between the second and third fingers, and the stain was so ingrained that no pumice could remove it. So here was something that they had shared.

For their copper wedding anniversary, my father had presented Germaine with a silver cigarette case with the engraving "Happy anniversary, my darling Germa, with love forever from your Mick." The gift was so dear to her that I decided to give her a lighter and cigarette holder to complement it. It was a great success: Germaine was clearly moved, and she thanked me effusively.

That evening we went to our old haunt, the Café Eylders, and as usual after dinner she went to smoke a cigarette. No longer was Mick there, of course, to take a cigarette from the case, light it, and lean forward to place it between her lips. I could not take the place of her husband. But I looked on with satisfaction as she took the cigarette from her precious case and placed it in the holder, lighting it with her new lighter.

As we prepared to leave, she opened her bag and was just dropping the holder inside when a voice came from the next table.

"Oh, madam, what a beautiful cigarette holder!"

The speaker was a girl; she was sitting with a boy about her own age, and they both looked rather poor. My mother smiled and handed the holder to her, as if to allow her to examine it more closely. The girl took it and turned it over in obvious admiration, then held out her hand to return it.

"No," said my mother. "Keep it. It has been very dear to me, but I want you to have it. And this is the matching lighter. They go together, so here, take it as well."

The girl blushed scarlet with embarrassment and shook her head, but Germaine pressed the lighter firmly into her hand.

"They are really smart—enjoy using them. Just mind they don't tempt you to smoke too much."

I was flabbergasted. A gift from her only child, chosen especially for her, given away without an instant's thought. Suddenly I seethed with impotent rage, with jealousy toward this unknown woman. Had my own mother chosen her over me?

Germaine seemed oblivious of my feelings. But now, many years later, I've come to realize that it couldn't have been rejection that was going through her mind. Her gesture came from the heart; there was hardly a moment for her to consider the consequences of her spontaneous generosity. Had she kept the gifts, I know well, they may have remained for years hidden away in some dark corner of a cupboard. My mother always took joy in giving; she enjoyed the idea that someone else might enjoy using them, and I find that quality of hers endearing.

THERE WERE MANY EVENINGS when I went out with friends, and I traveled quite a lot, so Germaine was often left to her own devices. In fact, she was a very lonely woman. After that desperate bout of drinking with Greet, the two women had drifted apart; Greet needed to devote her time to her husband, and that only made my mother's sense of loss more intense. No one could take Mick's place, but Germaine sorely needed a companion. Still, I was too absorbed by our own loving relationship to consider how lonely her hours without me must have been, and my mother was not one to complain.

One party to which I did bring my mother was a joint birthday celebration I staged with Mary Ann, a lesbian girlfriend of mine.

After my own matrimonial misadventures I equated monogamy with monotony, but unlike my relationship with Mary Ann, most of my affairs were heterosexual. So nearly all of my hundred or so guests were attractive, interesting, even eccentric, but straight, while Mary Ann brought about fifty birds of an altogether different plumage. They were mostly young and pretty girls who didn't flaunt their sexual orientation, so predictably some of my gallants with roving eyes made dates that proved disappointing.

A friend of mine owned the Okshoofd, a restaurant-cum-discotheque, and in return for the increased bar business he gave us exclusive use of the building and its garden for the night. I took my mother and some friends in my car, but there were several trays of food that had to be delivered to the Okshoofd, so I asked another lesbian friend, Hetty, to oblige.

Hetty and I had met shortly after my return from Canada, and I warmed to her at once. She was one of those good-natured, big-hearted women who was always ready to oblige. If somebody needed picking up from the airport or had heavy packages to collect, Hetty would be there without fail. I also liked her sense of fun; she was a regular patron of lesbian haunts like Homolulu, where the odd husband and wife sometimes dropped by to pick up a willing lesbian for a threesome session.

Having delivered the food, Hetty came over to be introduced to my mother, who was seated in regal splendor in a tall rattan chair. In contrast to Germaine's sober, elegant attire, Hetty sported a bright red jacket over a black-and-white-checked blouse. Hetty suffered from crippling rheumatism, and the pressure of a conventional handshake was agonizingly painful, but she took my mother's wrist and gave it a gentle squeeze.

"Hi, my name is Hetty. I'm a lesbian. What's your name, may I ask?"

Was Germaine reminded of Mick de Vries, of the forthright way he had announced his intention to marry her at their first meeting? Her response was similarly frigid. "My name is Germaine, and I am

Xaviera's mother. Your sexual preferences are of no interest to me. Now, would you please bring me a glass of medium dry sherry?"

Mary Ann and I were kept busy tending to our guests, and there was no way I could leave early to take my mother home. But Hetty never left her side for a moment during the entire evening, except for a few trips to the bar to replenish Germaine's glass or plate, she seemed drawn to her like a moth to flame. So when I suggested she might like to drive my mother home, Hetty was eager to oblige.

"Oh, and at the same time, could you drop off those boxes of fish salad, Hetty?" I called as they left. "We won't be needing them after all."

I have never asked either of them what they talked about during the drive back, but for Hetty, at any rate, the conversation must have been fascinating. This became evident about a week later when she drove over and mentioned there was a ghastly pungent smell in her car.

"I noticed it a day or two ago, but I have no idea what it can be, and I've been too busy to do anything about it." We opened the trunk, and there were the forgotten boxes of rotten stinking fish.

By then, I had the impression that Germaine may have been as preoccupied as Hetty. She had called me a few days after the party. "Xaviera, tell me something about these lesbians. And this friend of yours, Hetty: what sort of a woman is she?" Her tone was matter-of-fact, without any hint of emotional interest.

"She's a good, honest-to-goodness woman. Maybe you should see a bit more of her; she would be good company for you. She could do with some companionship too. You see, just about the time Pappi died, Hetty's lover died of cancer; all her rushing about to parties is just a cover for her loneliness. You could go out together, visit places and see new faces. She's an excellent driver, and she never drinks. You could trust her; she is absolutely loyal."

I wondered about my mother's sudden interest in Hetty but thought no more about it. Then, the next day, I happened to drop in on my mother unannounced. I let myself in with my key and walked down the hall. There were women's voices in the kitchen, and I saw through the opaque glass of the top half of the door, two silhouettes. One had to be my mother; the other was shorter. I opened the door and walked in.

There was Hetty, standing on tiptoe, with one arm around Germaine's waist, stroking her hair and reaching to kiss her lips. It was a moment of exquisite tenderness, but I was thunderstruck. Startled at my sudden appearance, Germaine hastily withdrew from Hetty's embrace. In a daze of disbelief I turned on my heel, hurried out of the apartment and into my car, and drove home.

I was still in a state of shock as I came through the front door. The phone was ringing.

"Veraatje, please don't think ill of me," Germaine implored. "You must understand, it was Hetty who made the move. She went to kiss me. You *know* me. You must know I'm not like that."

Qui s'excuse, s'accuse, or, as the Germans say, *Wer sich verteidigt klagt sich an:* he who excuses himself confesses. "Please, Mom, just give me time to get things straight in my mind. I need to let things sink in."

AND THAT WAS the beginning of a relationship that would last for twenty years. Though they became inseparable, both women kept their own apartments; Germaine would protest that the butchy gray-haired woman at her side was merely a good friend and companion who also happened to do her housekeeping. For all those years, she could never bring herself to utter the word *lesbian*. And Hetty would swallow her pride and agree with anything she said.

I caught on quickly. Hetty always relished greeting each new day with a bright new outfit, so when I looked in on my mom one day and saw Hetty there in the slacks and blouse I knew she'd worn the day before, it was clear where she'd slept that night. A few days later I noticed some of her clothes hanging in my mother's closet; later I discovered her toothpaste in the bathroom.

At first I felt jealous once again, as it became obvious that Hetty adored Germaine. In my bitterness, I recalled a conversation I'd had with Germaine only a year or so earlier. She had been seeing a very handsome man, an architect, and he had actually gone so far as to propose to her. But she was having none of it.

"No, Xaviera, I just cannot love this man the way I loved Mick. Besides, the time is past for me to start looking after a man's needs again. For thirty years I washed and ironed Mick's clothes, arranged them every night, cooked for him, and helped him in his practice. And then there were all those years I tended him through his illness. I'm tired, and I'm getting too old to start romancing a man all over again. I must learn to live on my own, and look after myself."

Yet she also added: "Perhaps someday I shall find someone who will look after me. That would be the perfect situation."

So perhaps, I thought, Hetty's arrival would prove a blessing. And besides, who was I, who had slept with so many men and women, to be so easily shocked? I hated hypocrites; was I turning into one myself? And who had brought these two women to-gether? They were both lonely and unhappy, and it wasn't as though a woman would compete with the memory of my father. I don't think I could have accepted another man. Hetty, on the other hand, had so much in common with Germaine. Coming from the south of the country, she had something of the vivacity Germaine had inherited from her French mother. Cologne, the home of Germaine's father, was a carnival city, as was Hetty's birthplace. Hetty was an enthusiastic photographer, a hobby that Germaine also enjoyed. If she couldn't match my father's scholarly bent, so what? Hetty's warmth and uncomplicated affection could prove to be exactly what Germaine needed.

As the years passed, I came to realize how fond Hetty was of me. And it was to me that she would turn when she found Germaine cold or unresponsive. One day she sought me out in my kitchen for consolation. "Why can't she just tell me she loves me?" she demanded. "She can be so formal—so German!"

My mother never displayed her emotions in public, I explained. Even in intimate moments, her manners were often reserved. And in her last years, age and illness did render Germaine's moods more difficult to cope with. Hetty understood and shared my mother's suffering, but still she sometimes found her behavior hard to bear.

"She just won't say such things," I answered. "I guess you'll just have to *feel* her love. Some people are just less able than others to express what goes on in their hearts."

"Xaviera, if I didn't love you so much as a friend, I couldn't put up with Germaine's stories much longer. She never stops worrying about you. All she ever talks about are you, the good times she and Mick had together, and the horrors of the prison camp."

I had a lot of sympathy for Hetty. In the years after Mick's death Germaine had been deserted by a number of women she'd regarded as friends but who now saw this still-attractive widow as a potential threat. Hetty, for her part, took pains to adapt her way of life to please Germaine. She couldn't completely eradicate her butch appearance, but she took great care over her long, polished fingernails and cut off her ponytail to make my mother feel more comfortable. And she never took advantage of Germaine's generous nature. Although she had left home and quit school to be able to live her lesbian life without shaming her affluent family, they had never rejected her. So when she came to live with Germaine, she owned a house in the country as well as her Amsterdam apartment, had her own car, and received a monthly allowance that assured her independence.

The last years of my mom's life brought her much pain and suffering, but she was spared the desolation of loneliness.

22

New Horizons

MURRAY WAS a soft-spoken man in his midforties, a lover and good friend from my days in Canada. I think he was always keener on golf than on business, but he'd been sufficiently successful in the latter for him to retire and indulge his passion for the former. He was drawn to settle in Andalucía by the prospect of long sunny days on the magnificent courses that dot this stretch of the Spanish coast. Here he was able to enjoy his eighteen holes in shorts and T-shirt, very different from his customary costume in Thunder Bay.

When he learned I was back in Europe, Murray got in touch. "You should come here for a vacation," Murray suggested. "You always loved the sun, and there's plenty going on in Marbella. Just let me know when you or any of your friends would like to visit, and I'll show you around."

I didn't feel like going myself just then, but I thought my mother might enjoy a break. She was always giving me presents; here was an opportunity for me to give something back. I knew I could trust Murray to look after her and see that she enjoyed herself. So off she went. Murray was at Málaga Airport to meet her, but at the sight of him she recoiled in horror.

"When I saw that gray-haired man standing there, I thought it was Larry," she told me when she phoned. "I remembered the way he used to steal from you in New York. I was terrified that you were going to get into trouble again."

Until that moment I'd never noticed the resemblance between the two men, but she was right. I had long forgiven Larry for his pilfering, and we were once again on friendly terms. But my mother remained deeply suspicious, of him and any other new man who crossed my path. She was only too aware of my gullibility: in my time I've fallen for quite a few smooth talkers, and Germaine's nightmare was that one day I would wake up and find myself penniless. (She needn't have worried; for all my flights of fantasy, I've always had a core of good, old-fashioned Dutch hardheadedness.)

Germaine took quite a fancy to Marbella. The climate was good, which would later be a comfort to arthritic Hetty, and there were elegant shops and a sizeable Dutch community to make her feel at home. When she was ready for another visit, I decided to take up Murray's offer and join her for a short holiday myself. I would end up making the place my second home for twenty years.

One of the first people I met was David, a former merchant banker in his midfifties who had left England after what he called a "difference of opinion" with Her Majesty's Treasury. There was an immediate rapport between us: both of us had been uprooted and were being forced to start an entirely new life. He was in the process of buying an apartment in Puerto Banus, a new development on the coast, a dozen kilometers outside Marbella. These days Puerto Banus is a trendy, crowded resort for the rich and glamorous; back then it was a quiet, intimate little huddle of shops and apartments overlooking a small harbor. I liked his new home, a studio in exquisite taste, and it gave me the idea of buying a place of my own. But I wanted something bigger where I could entertain friends, or invite my mother and Hetty for a vacation, and I definitely wanted it in town. So I bought an apartment on the fourth floor of a tall, rather impersonal block as a pied-à-terre. Balconies on two sides relieved the starkness of the building, one giving a view of the sea, the other of busy streets—the contrasting aspects of Marbella that attracted relaxation, activity, and me.

The apartment proved a great success with my friends, and after a while I found I was spending more and more time there. So when the penthouse became available, I literally traded up. I brought a lot of my personal possessions from Holland and bought new furniture and appliances. What started as a holiday hideout turned into a home.

Things like stereo systems and kitchen appliances were expensive and heavily taxed in Spain, yet just over the horizon Gibraltar beckoned with streets full of tax-free shops. After visiting David one day, I strolled through the marina and came across Dirk, the brawny Dutch skipper of a fast motor launch. He made no secret of his profession, smuggling cigarettes and alcohol from Gibraltar. With its passages through the apartment blocks leading to the street, Puerto Banus could have been designed for smuggling: it was simply a matter of driving away, bypassing the customs check at each end of the marina. Dirk found a convenient date, we agreed on a price, and David and I hired him and his craft for a two-day shopping expedition.

The day before we were to sail, Dirk called me to say the trip was off. I asked the reason, but he was evasive; I figured some more profitable offer had turned up. I was furious, but he told me to calm down: the boat next to his could be hired instead. So David and I boarded a former landing craft bought after the war by Adrian, another Englishman like David. He and his girlfriend, Becky, were ready and willing to accept a charter: neither they, nor their slightly decrepit boat, suggested affluence.

We set out together, noting without surprise that Dirk's berth was already empty. Our progress was leisurely: if Dirk's boat was a greyhound, then Adrian's resembled an aged, slightly lame sheepdog. But the company was pleasant, and when we weren't admiring the view of the Spanish coast, we feasted our eyes on Becky, who had posed as a model for Cinzano TV ads. The harbor at Gibraltar was packed with every kind of boat, and our launch attracted no attention when it limped alongside a quay. But the following day, when we returned, I was alarmed to see the quay lined with Spanish police as we approached Adrian's berth. Our cabin was crammed with contraband in cardboard cartons, and on deck stood a scooter I had bought, plain as day. Oh God, I thought, after all the trauma I've had with the law in the States and Canada, now I have to get in trouble in Spain!

Adrian looked grim, but he was ready to save us if he could. "As soon as we're moored, you two jump ashore and walk away as though there's nothing wrong. I'll stay behind to talk to the reception committee, try to bluff my way out of this mess. If we manage to get away with it, I'll deliver your stuff to David's apartment after dark. Sorry, Xaviera, but you may have to wait a day or two for the scooter. I can say it belongs to the boat, and I am going to license it during the week."

We made fast next to Dirk's still-empty berth, and David and I clambered ashore, trying to look like we ran into gangs of police every day of the week. They were oblivious. They never gave us a glance and ignored Adrian and his boat altogether. We sauntered off the quay, relieved but puzzled. That evening Adrian brought our goods to David's apartment.

"How'd you make out?" I asked.

"No problem. They weren't interested in us. The moment Dirk got back from Morocco, they were all over his boat. Turns out they've been watching him for months."

Obviously there was more money to be made shipping drugs

than cigarettes, which explained Dirk's last-minute cancellation of our charter. But the penalty if you got caught was that much harsher: I never saw Dirk or his boat again.

I WASN'T the only person buying things for my new homes in Amstelveen and Marbella. Germaine delighted in showing her love by giving me practical presents. She had impeccable taste—but unfortunately it wasn't the same as mine. When I decided I needed a new carpet, I had my heart set on cream or gray: she bought me a pure white one that would show up every mark. The table lamp she gave me would have been fine, if only the table had been wide enough to hold it. She even bought me new curtains that worked just fine, but their purple velour seemed more suitable for a funeral parlor than my living room. I was too touched by her generosity to question her. Although she had sufficient means, now that she was a widow without an income I insisted on giving her a monthly allowance, and I was unhappy that she should spend it buying things for me.

After some years, though, I hit upon the idea of giving her and Hetty something she couldn't return to me: a holiday in New York. I called two friends from my swinging days—Ted, a wealthy businessman, and Peter, my lawyer—who I knew would pull out all the stops to make sure the two elderly ladies had a great time from the moment they arrived. At the airport they were escorted to Ted's stretch limousine and driven to his home on Fifth Avenue: a gigantic and luxurious apartment resplendent with priceless antique furniture, the walls hung with fine delicately colored paintings. They were wined and dined by their host, and then given the run of the place as Ted and his wife moved out for two weeks to their place in the Hamptons. They had everything they could desire: from daily newspaper delivery and multichannel TV to a Jacuzzi, which they seemed to have found too daunting to use. I never asked whether they understood the purpose of the huge cushions scattered all over the rooms, or the bed that could be adjusted into any position. But they certainly appreciated the arrival of the maid each morning, bringing them a breakfast of scrambled eggs, fresh coffee, and fruit juice in bed.

Having visited me while I was working in New York, my mother had become accustomed to my New York apartment, which had been even more lavish than Ted's. But this was a totally new experience for Hetty, who was quite overwhelmed. In Amsterdam the very practical Hetty, who looked after Germaine, could enjoy the feeling that she was in charge. Now, though, the roles were reversed. To Hetty everything was new and exciting, as though she were a kid on her first outing, while Germaine carried herself with the self-assurance of a widely traveled woman comfortable in the most sophisticated circles. Hetty's sense of dependence was all the greater because of Germaine's fluent English; Hetty, who'd had little formal education, was hopeless at languages. Throughout the trip Germaine was reminded of the way Mick had shown her around Paris: he had been the great teacher to her assiduous pupil, and now she easily assumed his role with her companion.

During the day Germaine and Hetty enjoyed the wonders of window-shopping at its brightest and best, before being picked up by Peter for dinner at Sardi's, the fashionable restaurant in the theater district. The women were impressed by the glamour of their surroundings. "Is there nobody in New York over fifty?" Germaine asked.

Peter laughed. "Welcome to the Land of Eternal Youth. Haven't you ladies ever heard of plastic surgery?"

Hetty squinted at a woman at the next table, an exotic seventy-year-old who had undergone the full treatment, and was amazed at not being able to find a single scar. What a contrast to Germaine, who had never given a thought to erasing her own age lines.

By the time they had disposed of their rich meals and a bottle of fruity California zinfandel, the years seemed to have slipped away from the women, as had their inhibitions.

"Now you're not going to tell me that *that* woman has been arti-ficially rejuvenated." Germaine giggled, nodding toward a dazzling blonde at a nearby table.

"No," Peter agreed. "That's the real thing. Her escort is a wealthy banker, a client of my firm. Most of his girlfriends are less than half his age."

"But he has a great head of hair," commented Hetty. "Men don't go bald here either?"

"Well, we men are just as vain as the ladies. He may have had a hair transplant—he can afford it. Or perhaps a well-fitting toupee. And the guys who run salons—you wouldn't believe what they can do here with a few sparse tufts of gray hair. It gets fixed, fluffed, interwoven, dried, sprayed, brushed, and combed until it looks like an eighteen-year-old's."

"And it lasts?" Hetty asked.

"Sure—until the guy jumps into a pool or meets up with a sud-den gust of wind."

Germaine looked thoughtful but said nothing. As they were leaving, though, she turned to Peter and thanked him profusely for everything he'd done. "But now I want to ask you one more favor."

"Go right ahead."

"May I pull your hair—not too hard, just enough to prove it's yours?"

Hetty blushed scarlet, but Peter roared with laughter. "Tug as hard as you like. It's all my own. My father still had his thick white thatch on the day he died, and he was ninety-two!"

They were still joking and fooling around when Peter put them in a cab and sent them home. As she told me later, Hetty had been eyeing Germaine keenly throughout the evening: though the two women had now lived together harmoniously for several years, she knew Germaine was still a man's woman, with a flirtatious streak that could still make her want to touch a man—even if only to pull his hair.

They spent the rest of their trip bustling blissfully about, travel-

ing to the Hamptons, exploring shops and museums, looking up
friends whose addresses I had given them. One area I told them to
avoid was Times Square, not a safe district in those days for a couple of elderly ladies on their own. But there was a devil in Hetty
that urged her to stroll through the sleazy part of town. So, against
her better judgment, Germaine agreed to stop down through what
was then the sex center of the city—with Hetty, the photo fiend,
carrying her new video camera in an open bag.

At one point a boy brushed up against my mother, then called
out to tell her she had bloodstains on her white coat. She looked
down and saw a spot but had no idea how it got there. The kid
insisted on being helpful, led them into a sex shop, and asked the
shopkeeper to get some water to sponge the stain. He grumbled
but went to the back of the shop and returned with a bowl of water
and a towel. Hetty had put her bag down on the counter while she
sponged the stain, which disappeared very quickly. When she
looked around, the helpful youth had disappeared too—along with
her video camera and, according to the furious shopkeeper, a batch
of porn videos.

When they told me the story, I explained that the "blood" was
just ketchup, and that they'd fallen for one of the oldest scams in
the book. I scolded Hetty for being so stupid—after all, she'd been
warned—but she was unrepentant.

"What's all the fuss?" she demanded. "It was insured for more
than it was worth. I've already bought a much better one with the
money, faster and lighter."

All she'd lost was the footage of their time in New York.

IT WAS IRONIC that I was able to present them with this welcome to America even as I myself was still forbidden to enter the
country. On one occasion I was even refused entry to England by
an overzealous immigration officer when I arrived with my mother
for a shopping expedition. His action was illegal: there was no

international warrant issued against me, and being Dutch I was perfectly entitled to enter any of the European Union countries. But the experience so upset Germaine that I never pursued the matter.

But America was different. Not only did I have many friends in the United States, but there were also lots of unscrupulous characters there, happily exploiting my name in my absence. There was a mediocre movie called *The Happy Hooker Goes to Washington*, shot without any attempt to contact me, and pirated editions of my books were on sale in bookstores all over the world. My hopes rose when NBC appealed to the State Department on my behalf, as they wanted me to appear on the *Today* show. But they were refused, and Tom Snyder and the full TV crew were obliged to fly to Paris to interview me in the Hotel George V.

The height of absurdity was reached a few years later, when the Justice Department demanded I be subpoenaed to appear as a witness in their case against an architect who had dodged taxes by pretending that my girls had been his employees. I didn't owe him anything, and I was ready to testify if they'd have me. But the State Department overruled the Justice Department and persisted in refusing me entry, even for a day or two, to allow me to appear in court. Perhaps if Clinton had been president then, I might have been allowed in; for that matter, I might have been invited to a private meeting in the White House!

Eventually, though, even the most bigoted and unreasonable so-called moralists were obliged to relent. After all, I was appearing constantly as a guest speaker at colleges and universities all over the globe. I was welcomed as a participant in sexology congresses in Mexico City and Jerusalem, along with highly respectable academics. On vacation I was even allowed to pass into Hungary and the former Czechoslovakia with no problem. So were Communist dictatorships more liberal than the United States, the Land of the Free?

Eventually I was granted a visa for a limited period, with all kinds of restrictions, to give some lectures and appear on TV. Only after it became apparent that my presence posted no threat to the national welfare was I able once more to come and go as I pleased.

WHAT MATTERED TO ME more than entry to any country was being accepted by my mother. To save her embarrassment, for more than ten years I had refused to authorize a Dutch edition of *The Happy Hooker*. It was enough of a shock for her to learn that her daughter had become the queen of the American sex industry, without having my face staring out at her in every bookstore. To her credit, she never condemned me or complained about what anyone else would think. If at first she reacted with silence, almost disbelief, nevertheless she stood by me with love and loyalty. By the time she and Franny were marching their Wellington boots through the Toronto mud, she was able to see the humor in the situation, and she even took a quiet pride at my success as the author of "that book."

Then Hetty came into her life, and she saw how her former prejudices had blinded her to so much simple joy. Now this conservative woman, who had burned my adolescent diary, read *The Happy Hooker,* at last available in Dutch.

"Why didn't anyone write a book like this thirty years ago, when Mick and I were getting married?" she asked.

"Because nobody was allowed to write honestly about sex," I replied. "A book like that would have gotten publisher and author alike burned at the stake."

"But now I finally understand: all those things Mick wanted me to do, which I thought were somehow dirty or perverted, were just innocent foreplay, something to stimulate the fantasy life of a husband for his wife. You know, when we were young there weren't even porno films; there wasn't even a *Penthouse* or *Playboy*. Now it's all discussed out in the open, even on TV. If your book had been around then, there would have been far fewer relationship problems."

But I wasn't sure about that. Even with all this new permissiveness and promiscuity, I wondered aloud whether something valuable may have disappeared. When there were still taboos, I had the wonder of discovering my own secrets, exploring the hidden landscape of a boyfriend's body, even while I hung on to my own virginity. Where's the magic when a mother gives her fifteen-year-old son a box of condoms, or gives her fourteen-year-old daughter the pill? Kids need to do things in their own time, I think. In my youth, we rebelled against our lack of liberty. Today's kids are rebelling against something different: having liberty thrust on them by well-meaning but inconsiderate parents.

Having finally won my mother over to my way of thinking, could it be that I was now the one who was standing up for old-fashioned values?

23

"There Are No Rules:
Expect the Unexpected"

"MISS HOLLANDER, my name is Dr. Gerhard Schlesinger. Like yourself, I am a professional writer, largely of erotica. I have been invited by the editor of *Der Stern* to submit an article for the magazine based on interviews with you. Your memoirs made you the most celebrated author on the real-life experience of the sex industry, and *Der Stern* is the largest-circulation magazine in Germany. So will you permit me to visit you in Amsterdam?"

The voice on the phone was quiet and cultured, and I was intrigued to find out what sort of man Dr. Schlesinger was in the flesh. We consulted our calendars, and a few days later I picked him up at Schiphol and took him home. I had by now outgrown my Amstelveen home and bought a substantial house in the heart of Amsterdam, a much more suitable place in which to put up such visitors as Dr. Schlesinger, who proved to be the epitome of courtesy.

He knew my *Penthouse* column, in both English-language and German versions, and I learned that he wrote a series of witty articles under the pseudonym Felix Freitag. Somehow the name suited him; from then on he was always Felix to me. He was an attractive man, intellectual but unpretentious, and undoubtedly sexy. I was very ready to cooperate with him, both on the page and between the sheets. His visits to Amsterdam became a regular habit; later he returned my hospitality by arranging for me to write a piece on the nightlife of Hamburg, his native city, where he showed me around, introduced me to everybody, and generally looked after me.

From the outset, though, I was worried about how Germaine would take to this latest man in my life. When she disliked one of my partners, or even a casual acquaintance, the atmosphere could grow positively chilly. She was happy enough that I was a sought-after author, but was very hostile to any suggestion that the Happy Hooker was still in business. So even interviews for as influential a journal as *Der Stern* could provoke anxiety that I might still be reliving my past.

Felix had the advantage of being able to speak with my mother in her own native tongue, with the accent of an educated scholar; that alone inspired a degree of confidence. But he was so debonair that I think he would have won her over in any language. From their first meeting he never failed to bring flowers for her as well as for me. He was extremely well read, very musical, and each time he visited he invited me to a concert or a ballet—respectable outings of which Germaine couldn't help but approve.

Of course there were other performances of which my mother remained unaware. I had for some time become as much interested in the doings of my partners' minds as the doings of their bodies: particularly under the influence of mild hallucinogenic drugs, inhibitions disappeared and inner fantasies emerged from the depths of their subconscious. Sometimes I felt I was getting to know them better than they knew themselves, and I recorded their self-revelations on cassettes. Of course I proposed such a session to Felix: we would both consume magic mushrooms, so the result would be a mind-blown conversation, not a monologue. He had never taken mushrooms, but he agreed, trusting me to administer a safe dose.

I had noticed how scrupulously Felix used to remove any solitary hair he found on his chest with a pair of golden tweezers. Although he exhibited no trace of homosexual appetites, I was sure I detected a feminine cast to his personality, and it was this I was eager to explore.

After a light meal, I disconnected the doorbell and phones, opened the terrace door to let in the warm, scented air, and put on an extended tape of Chopin nocturnes. Then I switched on the recorder, and Felix settled down in a big leather easy chair. After a while, his customary, easy flow of talk dried up. He started becoming uncomfortably warm, so I suggested he slip into something more comfortable. I went upstairs and brought down a beautiful black silk gown from my bedroom closet, along with a string of pearls and a soft scarf. I ordered him to undress and put these on. Eased into a state of compliance, even docility, he undressed obediently in a corner of the living room, his back toward me. I noted with a smile that the briefs he had been wearing were a pair of my own.

Now, swathed in the soft folds of my gown, he permitted me to brush his thick mop of black hair so that it fell almost to shoulder length, very different from his habitual style. Before my eyes he was gradually transformed into a beautiful mature woman. It dawned on me that he was becoming a younger version of his mother, whom I had met.

We talked for hours, but when I attempted to commit what I term "tape rape"—seductively insinuating my impressions into his mind—he softly rebuffed my advances. "Xaviera, your mushrooms can take away my physical capabilities but not my mental ones."

And that got to the heart of our soul-searching expedition, together yet apart—a trip never to be forgotten, followed by a night of total loving.

EVER SINCE my mother admitted she had read *The Happy Hooker* and even approved of its message, a new intimacy had begun to grow up between us. The days of hiding my diary were long past; now, rejoicing in this openness, I played her the tape of my evening with Felix. She entered fully into the spirit of our mental striptease, and from then on she shared many such records (on tape or film) of intimate moments between me and my lovers—things I could share with no one else. I gave them to her to hide and secretly enjoy, first making sure that none was actually obscene or too shocking. So my mother came to share vicariously in her daughter's pleasures: just as Felix had regressed into his mother, my mother was beginning to share elements of my experience.

I got to know many different facets of Felix's character. A philosophy graduate, he had also become a devout Buddhist—disciplines that no doubt helped him endure my lengthy shopping sprees in patient silence. Always punctual, he was precise to the point of pedantry but never boring. Sophisticated and witty, he was a lively conversationalist; it was a delight for me to engage him in batting around topics of every stripe. And he was a sensual and accomplished lover.

So when it came, disenchantment was quite a shock. We had spent a week attending the World Congress of Sexology in Israel. Each night we made exquisite love together. But was something missing? I asked him to describe what he felt about me.

"Ach, Ich mag dich sehr gern!" he answered: I like you a lot.

I was stunned by the coolness. "I like *ice cream* a lot," I retorted. "What I feel for people close to me, even those who are no more than good friends, is love. I need passion in a lover, not indifference."

Felix spoke from the head. I needed a man who would shout from his heart. And two months later I met John Drummond.

I WAS SITTING on a restaurant terrace in Marbella with my old friends David and Franny, who'd flown in from New York for an ecstatic reunion with me. The evening was pleasantly cool and

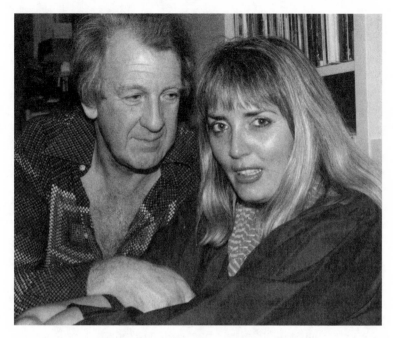

With John Drummond

relaxing after the blazing heat of a midsummer day. The waiter had just brought our meal when an apparition passed before my eyes. He took one look at the crowded terrace and slowly walked on. He was in his early fifties, tall and well built with a mop of unruly blond hair, casually dressed and wearing a contented smile. Instantly I knew that this would be the new man in my life.

Yet for one dread minute, having only just set eyes on him, I feared that he was walking straight out of my life again. Why did he then turn around and enter the restaurant? It was hunger, he said later. It was late, and most restaurants had stopped serving food. I'm convinced it was my psychic energy: I was certainly willing him to approach with all my might. There was one troubling moment when a waiter told him there was no table available, but he ignored the protest, walked inside, and ordered his food in fluent Spanish.

Returning to the terrace, he took a seat at a table that had just come available close to ours. The waiter insisted the table was reserved, only to be informed that it was now unreserved. The waiter cleared the table in defeat and brought him a bottle of red wine, but in removing the cork he managed to spill a quantity over his guest's white trousers. There followed the obligatory pantomime: profuse apologies and a mopping-up operation with towels and napkins. I saw my chance and took it.

Leaving David to look after Franny, I walked across and asked in English if he was alone, and if I might join him. Guessing he might be Scandinavian, I spoke clearly and deliberately, but I needn't have worried: he introduced himself as John Drummond, in the classic tones of an upper-class Englishman. Later I learned that his father was Scottish and his mother Russian, but for me he still is the archetypal upper-class English bohemian.

It turned out that we'd met fleetingly once before, about five years earlier, but since at the time he'd been with an extremely possessive woman, I hadn't paid any attention to him. But tonight John had noticed me and was already half in love with me without our exchanging a word. By the time he'd finished his steak, we were on sufficiently intimate terms for me to plunder his dessert while he was caressing my breasts. I loved the touch of his strong hands.

Naturally, when he had finished his meal I asked him to join us at my table. David took an instant liking to John; Franny, on the other hand, hated every moment of our flirtatious behavior and saw the rest of her vacation flash before her eyes, ruined by this interloper. I ordered Franny and David to take a taxi home, and whispered in David's ear that he should comfort Franny in his bed so John and I could carry on with our evening guilt-free.

We headed to a nearby bar for a nightcap and a most animated conversation, studded with tart English witticisms. I invited him back to my place for coffee, and offered to drive him, as he'd been drinking all evening. He accepted the coffee but refused the lift, explaining that his driving actually improved when he was a trifle drunk. A *trifle?* That was the understatement of the year. "If a man can't drive drunk," he argued, "he can't drive sober." So I got into my BMW, and he followed me in his beat-up Mini Cooper. He chased me all over town; when finally I decided to stop at a red light, I looked over to see him suddenly standing beside my open window, bellowing at the top of his voice: *"¡Yo te quiero!"* I love you!

That was how I wanted to be loved, with crazy exuberance. It was the beginning of a new life.

24

Don Juan

JOHN, who worked as a set designer in the movie industry, owned a *finca*, an unostentatious farmstead, in the hills just outside Mijas. At the time a quiet village, Mijas was soon to become an attraction for golf and tennis devotees and tourists, attracted in part by the pack of donkeys that roamed the streets masquerading as taxis, each bearing a license number. John's home had no such pretensions: primitive in its amenities, it was not my sort of place at all. I had grown used to driving on roads, not a dirt track; water running from a tap, not hauled up from a well. As for electricity, his ancient generator ought to have been stored away in a museum. My only consolations were a full-size bathtub and bidet, conveniences that looked quite out of place. For company he had a flock of chickens, resident pigeons, and a pointer, an English hunting dog with soulful eyes. But John was above all highly practical; he knew how to fix anything, and the place gave him security and independence. And he had set down roots in the area: he was a genuine local, with friends among the shopkeepers and a membership at La Cepa, his favored bar down on the coast at Fuengirola.

From the first days, and nights, we passed in each other's company John and I recognized that we belonged together. This was no passing encounter: even in our frequent, boisterous squabbles we brought each other to life, the air crackling with the electricity that flashed between us. My visits to Spain grew longer; John had grown so accustomed to the Andalusian climate and way of life that he wilted in Amsterdam, but wild horses couldn't have dragged me to live in John's spartan *finca*. So I seized the opportunity to buy a villa high above Marbella where we could live together. Now I was free to entertain as lavishly as I did in Holland: guests could relax in the spacious gardens or by the pool, and there was enough space for us both to invite our cronies without getting in each other's hair.

I shall always be grateful to John for getting me out of the noise and pollution of the town and into the sweet fresh air of the country, with a garden and dogs of my own. Even the chickens came along to take up residence: maybe they lowered the tone of the villa, but even our most highfalutin guests never complained about the abundant supply of fresh eggs.

In no time John had converted the garage into a storage space—and a repair shop for about half a dozen Minis, mostly old jalopies that would now be considered antiques. Eventually even the street in front of our luxurious villa began filling with old cars, to the dismay of our yuppie neighbors.

Of course, my mom and her faithful companion were among our most special guests. I wondered how they would get on with John: he was so different from Felix and nearly all the other men they had met in my house in Amsterdam. John has a wonderful command of the English language, but when aggravated, or loosened up by a dram or two of Scotch, he can turn the air blue with a stream of good, old-fashioned Anglo-Saxon expletives—certain, I feared, to offend my mother's delicate sensibilities.

I needn't have worried. John was always on his best behavior around her, and she and Hetty both melted at his charm—so much that during my occasional verbal brawls with John they weren't shy about siding with him. This was taking approval a bit too far!

ONE RESPECT in which John and I were well matched was our sexual freedom. I hadn't escaped from a married routine to be condemned to monogamy without matrimony. John blasted most of my casual lovers as a bunch of pimple-faced kids—but who was I to argue? He was right: most of my lovers were half my age. Less amusing for me was his string of lovers, almost all holiday girls from England with high-pitched North Country voices and girly giggles. Not for nothing was "Don Juan" the Spanish name for "John." Yet our mutual infidelities merely added piquancy to our own lovemaking—especially when we were apart—and whatever our adventures, we always returned to each other.

Together, we were an explosive mixture: so much so that we decided to write a book together. *Happily Hooked* was a hilarious account of the first six months of our tempestuous love affair, chronicling what happens when two raving egomaniacs get addicted to each other's bodies and minds. We realized early that each of us needs a degree of social friction to come alive, and we delighted in the thrust and riposte of verbal slapstick. To an unwitting outsider, the experience could be alarming—"*Donner und Blitzen* are at it again!" I'm sure the neighbors thought more than once—but we loved it.

Still, there were encounters when our mutual goading spiraled out of control. One evening, John was standing by the fridge, screaming an endless stream of insults at me as he poured himself a glass of milk. I can't recall what I'd said or done to provoke his outburst, but suddenly I just couldn't stand it any longer. The windows were closed, and his tirade was bouncing off the walls of the house. I shouted to him to stop, that I couldn't bear it another

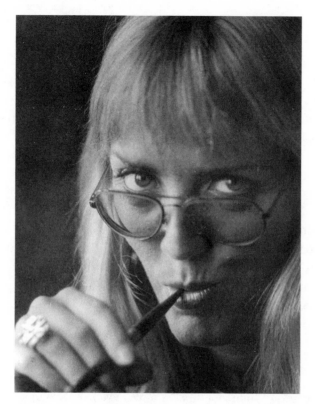

Pen at the ready

moment. But he knew he had the advantage, and only yelled all the louder. I could have killed him to shut his mouth—and impulsively grabbed a big, sharp kitchen knife from the rack. I almost thrust it into his back before a flash of reason took over. If in the morning his corpse had been discovered by our gardeners, I would have had a hard time explaining myself to them—after all, they were actually policemen who did a spot of gardening on the side.

Still, when John turned round and rested his hand on a wooden chopping board, I hurled the knife with all my might. It stood, quivering between his spread fingers, and he stared at it in horror and disbelief.

"What the fuck do you think you are doing?" he cried. "Good God, woman, you could have mutilated me!"

"You're lucky I didn't," I snapped. "You were driving me berserk. Now get the hell out of my kitchen—better still, out of my house!"

I must have scared the devil out of him. For once he didn't stop to argue but dashed straight out to his car. I heard him drive off, and finally the house was blissfully quiet—until he returned at three in the morning, his sorrows safely drowned.

The next morning, when Germaine and Hetty came by, they walked into the kitchen and saw the naked blade still firmly imbedded in the chopping board, fragments of its handle strewn on the floor. John followed them in and seized his opportunity.

"Your daughter tried to kill me. Just because she couldn't bear the sound of my cultured English voice," he told Germaine. He was speaking softly, in measured tones, but I could hear the sarcastic undertone.

My mom grimaced. "You had another of your mad attacks again," she accused me. "Why can't you get over your crazy fascination for knives!"

I turned to John in a fury. "You were yelling so loud you drove me mad! You did it on purpose. You knew you were provoking me, and you kept on even when I begged you to stop."

If I'd expected support from my mother, I was in for a disappointment. Ignoring me, she turned to John. "It's a streak of madness she gets from her father—something peculiar to people with Indonesian blood. They call it *mataglap*. Mick was the gentlest of men, but once when we were on holiday in Italy and some kid snatched my bag, he went after him so savagely it took four men to drag him off the thief. In everyday life he wouldn't have hurt a fly— but in the grip of that mad fury, he could easily have killed that man."

Hetty took control of the situation. "Come along, Xaviera," she said quietly. "You need to buy a new knife for your kitchen—that one's no good anymore. Let's go shopping." Turning to John, she added: "She must have had some good reason to lose her temper like that—I wouldn't try to make out that it was all her fault."

My own mother, siding with my man against me; her girlfriend taking my side. I took the two women with me into town and bought us all ice cream, figuring we all needed to cool down. Then Hetty and I left Germaine basking in the sunshine, and returned some time later with not one but three ferocious-looking kitchen knives. As soon as we got home, I resolved, I'd hide them away in a cupboard out of sight from my mother. The next time I flew into a tantrum in front of her, there'd better not be any knives nearby.

HETTY MAY HAVE SIDED with me against John on that horrendous occasion, but she and John usually got along quite well together—at least in small doses. Her masculine side showed in her delight in puttering about with every sort of gadget—something that appealed to John, the practical man about the house. When a video camera I had bought him for his birthday needed fixing, Hetty was able to teach him a trick or two—as I retreated to my computer to let the two technicians have their fun.

With Germaine, his relationship was more complex. He ribbed her frequently for never teaching me to be a proper housekeeper, spoiling me with maids to wait on me throughout my childhood. Then, when my fortieth birthday rolled around, my romantic lover announced that he'd bought me a very special gift. The package was carefully wrapped, but when I opened it I found only a box of aspirin and four Brillo pads. My mother could see I was upset but wisely held her tongue and smiled the incident off as a harmless joke.

Germaine was willing to forgive John much, for she knew there was another side to his character—a side that greeted me on another of my birthdays, when I drove from Amsterdam with Germaine and Hetty to meet him in Spain. Waiting for me there was a magnificent king-size bed he had painstakingly created for us, painting its every surface by hand with scenes from the *Kama Sutra*. The figures resembled John and me so closely that my mother seemed transfixed, gazing at the images of the intertwined lovers, doubtless remembering her own long-ago moments of bliss with her man. In some respects, my relationship with John resembled hers with Mick: at times she had argued with her husband as wildly as I did with John some mornings, at least until he had drained his first cup of coffee. Caffeine, like alcohol, stimulated him to fight back, and then we would go for each other, hammer and tongs.

But there were long, drowsy afternoons, with sun-shy Hetty busy inside with some piece of electronic equipment while John and Germaine chatted on the terrace almost like a couple of young lovers. All his boisterousness vanished, John would listen with infinite patience while she reminisced about the days before the war in Indonesia when she was the *nonja basar*—the great lady—and her husband the beloved and respected doctor. John surreptitiously refilled her sherry glass, making sure they were out of Hetty's sight, and in this mellow mood she laughed at his yarns but teared up at her own memories. She was just as emotional as her own mother had been, and John would put his arm around her and give her a gentle hug.

Although he showed me the same warm affection, he couldn't resist teasing me and having a joke at my expense. One boiling afternoon I had driven his dog to the vet, waiting for an eternity in the sweltering surgery before returning sticky, sweaty, and dying for a long cold drink. John was standing in the kitchen, about to drink a glass of fresh-squeezed orange juice, straight from the fridge.

"Let me have a sip of your juice," I pleaded.

"No, this is mine. You can damned well go and squeeze your own oranges."

I was outraged: after all, it was his damn dog I'd been suffering for all day. I let fly a torrent of abuse, but he only smiled in return, which of course drove me into wilder paroxysms of fury. And that was why as I was screaming I didn't notice that he'd switched on the cassette recorder he always kept in the kitchen. I carried on with my satisfying tirade, slamming the silverware drawer, finally resolving to make my own juice, and sulking around the house in resentment for a while until the storm passed.

A few days later, a particularly boring couple inflicted their presence on us and, despite my hints, remained oblivious to the fact that they'd outstayed their welcome. John, on the other hand, was being unusually polite to them, sitting them down and giving them a drink. At one point, as I sat inwardly fuming, John went to put on some music. Only it wasn't music: from the cassette recorder issued an unbroken stream of my howls of rage and curses, all reproduced in high fidelity and full volume. Our guests turned pale, glanced at each other in disbelief, and suddenly remembered they were due somewhere else.

Germaine was aghast. "Xaviera, how could you behave like that? It's disgusting. Please, John, turn it off."

But Hetty was laughing her head off. "No, keep it going. It's hilarious!"

"It's all right, Germaine," John assured her. "Xaviera was just getting a little overexcited, and I thought it'd be fun to get it down on tape—you know, for posterity."

I still have that cassette—and not just as a souvenir. You never know when it might come in handy again.

25

A Child No More?

LONG BEFORE my father died, I had grown out of my adolescent rivalry with my mother. Loving my father as I did, I came to admire the devotion with which she tended him in those last dreadful years, and that only enhanced my love for her. As a child I had wanted to be more like my father; now I began to relish Germaine's femininity, and to find things about her I yearned to emulate.

She had style, for one thing. Germaine took to the grave a knack for making herself look absolutely fabulous simply by wrapping a scarf around her neck in a certain way. Somehow, no matter how hard I tried, I could never quite figure out how she did it; she offered to show me dozens of times, but I was always running off with something else to do. Maybe that was what I wanted, that this should remain her own gift, rather than letting myself become a mere copycat of her inimitable chic.

I used to peep into her bedroom as she sat in front of the vanity, her beautiful face and slender neck reflected from every angle. She would get up from her dressing table and walk across to the

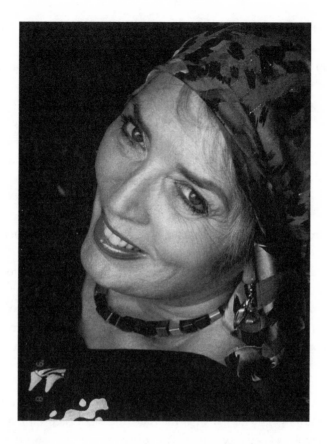

cabinet where she kept her wonderful collection of scarves of every hue in silk or crepe de chine, all stacked neatly or hanging from special hangers. From my earliest childhood, I can remember breathing in their aroma, watching with wonder as she selected the brooch and matching earrings without which she would never have left the house. As if by magic, her delicate fingers would transform a simple rectangle of material into a veritable work of art.

Sometimes I was allowed to choose her scarf, but among my fondest memories were the days when she placed one of her glorious scarves around my neck, taking me shopping or to visit friends. On occasion I was treated to lunch at the magnificent department store De Bijenkorf, and I felt myself the proudest kid in the block to be seen with such an attractive mother.

So strong did my own fetish for scarves become that I used to sneak into my mother's room and carry off one of hers whenever I was going on a trip abroad. Over the years, I must have lifted dozens from her collection, gradually building one of my own, like some obsessed lepidopterist amassing specimens. When I began earning serious money, I repaid her by buying her the most precious and exotic scarves I could find, from every corner of the earth.

My mother's touch of vanity remained until the very end of her life. She was eighty-three when I brought a couple of quite splendid scarves home for Christmas, intending to give one to her and the other to a friend who shared Germaine's taste in clothes. I gave the warmer of the two to my mother, but when she got a look at Lidewij's silkier present, an infantile pout came over her, and she demanded that one instead. My friend was only too willing to comply, and I tried to find what consolation I could in the idea that the strains of old age hadn't tempted my mother to let herself go.

GERMAINE AND I developed a ritual over the years. Provided I was not living with a man at the time, the night before I left for a holiday she would stay with me and drive me to the airport the next morning. And when I returned she would be waiting faithfully to help with my wealth of baggage and take me home again. Even in old age she retained her vigor; she could always outwalk me, and it was a joy to spot her in her bright shawl, holding a welcoming batch of flowers, with Hetty by her side. Whenever I could I traveled with my dogs, and they would rush to greet her, barking excitedly and jumping at her feet. And that first night after my return was sacrosanct: even Hetty would leave us alone as she brought me up to date with her news, and I shared my travel stories until, deliciously tired, we would go to bed and snuggle together, comforted by our warmth and closeness.

On one such occasion, we had just finished a tasty meal she'd cooked especially for me and I was preparing to unpack when there was a ring at the front door.

"Can't we just pretend there's nobody here?" pleaded Germaine.

"Mom, I can't leave somebody standing there without even knowing who it is."

"But this is our night," she said reproachfully. "I haven't seen you for nearly two months."

I wasn't expecting any visitors, but as I gazed at the great jumble of luggage it occurred to me that it would be nice to have a man there to help me. And *voilà!* Standing on my doorstep was George Goudsmit, an old school pal and former lover now living at the Findhorn Foundation in Scotland. From time to time he returned to Amsterdam to visit his ailing parents, but their house was small and depressing, and George usually spent a few nights with me in my master bedroom or in a guest room. He knew he was always welcome in my house—always, but not tonight.

Reluctantly, I let him in. My mother, who had always liked him, stared at him icily. Sensing the atmosphere, George followed me into the hall, where I explained the awkward situation. Fully aware of my mother's mood swings, he happily agreed to find a hotel for the night. Before he left, I gave him a kiss at the top of the stairs.

"Veraaaa! What's taking you so long?" called my mother.

I have never got rid of a friend so quickly—but not before getting him to lug my suitcases into the bedroom.

But there were other occasions when I was able to turn to my mother for company and consolation after showing a lover the door. Once I was delighted to have a visit from a handsome, sexy actor I hadn't seen for years. He'd just returned from a six-month sabbatical in Australia, and we prepared to celebrate our reunion with a night of bliss. I disconnected the phones and arranged the living room and bedroom with every temptation imaginable. Candles flickered; the air was heavy with incense, while some of his favorite music played softly in the background. Together we prepared a memorable meal; then, around midnight, we climbed the stairs for the rest of the evening. After sharing a hot, fragrant bath, we danced together before climbing into bed.

I had just taken him in my arms when he pulled away and told me he'd recently been married; his wife was about to have a baby, he said, and he was consumed with pangs of guilt. Then again, I thought in frustration, maybe he's just afraid his wife will return home unexpectedly and deduce that he's out with another woman. Whatever the reason, he jumped out of bed, struggled into his clothes, and fled.

In shock and misery I got up, put on a long, slinky nightgown— for nobody's benefit, alas—and wandered disconsolately downstairs. The candles were still burning, as if to mock my unhappiness.

I knew my mother suffered from insomnia; she rarely made it to sleep before about 3 A.M., and then only after taking sleeping pills. So I picked up the phone and called her. We were frequent phone partners during the day, but at this time of night she seemed to know I must be hurting before I even had time to tell her what had happened. Twenty minutes later I heard her car pull up outside.

I'd prepared some fruit salad for her and poured her a glass of sherry. She gave me a hug and looked anxiously into my eyes before asking what was wrong. As we settled down on a couch, she looked around in amazement.

"So this is what the place is like when you're in the mood for seduction." She smiled.

"You mean the candles and the music," I said innocently.

"I mean *everything*—even you yourself seem different. I never get to see you so mellow and radiant during the day; you're always on the phone or running off to a meeting. Now here you are, wearing makeup, looking so sexy . . . and alone?"

"Well, why do you think I called!"

"There was a man here? What happened—did he desert you?"

"You could put it that way," I answered.

"So what went wrong?"

I told her the whole story. "And then he had the nerve to tell me this naive young wife of his was insanely jealous! One sniff and she'd have known he'd been with another woman."

"Women do have that kind of intuition." Germaine sighed, doubtless thinking back to her own trials with Mick. "So what happened?"

"Nothing—absolutely nothing. He rushed out of the house, leaving me devastated. I needed someone to talk to. Would you hold me for a little while?"

She took my hand, and together we sank into the couch. I put my head on her shoulder and inhaled her sweet scent. Her face looked young and radiant again, her hair a little disheveled; she must have been in bed already when I called. So natural a look made her seem not quite the perfect lady—more like a young girl.

I got up to change the music, putting on Schubert's *Death and the Maiden* Quartet. I dived into the fruit salad, spoon-feeding Germaine the delicious chunks of mango, peach, strawberries, and pineapple. The candles burned down as we talked, and dawn was breaking before I led her upstairs and we climbed into bed. I had put on Beethoven's *Moonlight Sonata*, and my eyes filled with tears as we both remembered Pappi playing those very strains himself. My mother fell asleep with her head on my arm. We lay together, and then I too dropped into slumber, soothed by the gentle sound of her regular breathing.

PERHAPS WE NEVER CEASE being children. After my father's death, I was always attracted to men who reminded me of some element of his personality. I had affairs with younger men, often passionate and deeply emotional, but I was always vulnerable to the charisma of intellectual and artistic men much older than I, usually Jewish, to whom I could look for guidance or inspiration. I knew I would never find a reincarnation of my father, but I never stopped looking for him—a quest that led to some of my most profound friendships.

On the other hand, in my adolescent lesbian affairs with older women, I was rebelling against the authority of my mother and the control she tried to exercise over my conduct. Maybe too I was acting out my resentment that it was she who was my father's life partner. After his death, though, the new admiration I felt for my mother gave me a new perspective: without quite being aware of it, I began to be attracted by older women who seemed to share something of her charm. This child inside me now was looking for both her father and her mother among her lovers.

No one shared so many of my mother's traits as Mathilde, a woman some eighteen years my senior whom I met in Marbella while I was still living in the penthouse apartment. She had a full round face with bright, happy eyes. Her skin was soft, her ash-blond hair always immaculate; it was some time before I discovered it was a wig. Unlike my mother, though, Mathilde possessed two utterly different sides to her personality. Smartly dressed and beautifully made up, with her long, slender fingers and manicured red nails, she resembled Germaine in her elegance and femininity. When I could persuade her to cast aside her wig, however, she became another person: decidedly butch, a real tomboy.

On that first afternoon, though, as she welcomed me into her house for tea, it was I who was the tomboy. I'd come straight from the beach with sand between my toes, my flesh smelling of the salty sea. By contrast, everything about Mathilde had an air of refinement and that sense of German correctness she shared with Germaine. Theirs was a calm, methodical way of life, so different from my own frenzied pace. At first I was irritated by her insistence that I take off my sandy shoes before walking over her valuable Persian carpets, but as I looked around I realized her home merited respect: it was full of fine antique furniture—heirlooms, no doubt—and the walls were graced with stunning works of art.

She even ordered me to wash my hands before our meal of tea and tasty tidbits, all served in the most delicate fashion. Ravenous from my day in the sun, I wolfed down the food so fast that she had to tell me to slow down, warning me that if I didn't learn to moderate my eating, I'd develop a weight problem. *Yes, Mommy!*

As we ate, Mathilde told me her life story. For twenty years she'd been married to a wealthy businessman, which brought her financial security and respectability in the conservative village where she lived. But all the time she had been living a secret lesbian life, indulged in while working as a singer and entertainer on cruise ships. She showed me albums full of photographs of handsome male passengers who'd been her admirers, but smiled and sighed that she'd never fancied any of them. She had been attracted by the captains, but more by their wives, and the real highlight of the album was the pictures of beautiful young women who had been her lovers. In her turbulent youth she'd even been friendly with Marlene Dietrich. And there were photographs of Mathilde herself, a curvaceous, alluring young woman in long evening gowns, chic cocktail dresses, or white bathing suits that clung to her firm breasts. As I looked I began to feel a warm, glowing sensation inside me, the familiar desire to know more. She leaned over to brush the sand out of my hair, and I inhaled the aroma of her delicately scented body.

Slowly but deliberately, she set about her seduction. Lulled by the warmth of the summer evening and the contentment that follows an afternoon tea, I responded to her strong yet delicate fingers, to the fullness of those red lips that seemed both to promise and to threaten, and to the soft, low tones of her German voice. It was an unusual role for me: I had been a man's woman for quite a while, and it had been some time since I'd enjoyed more than a casual affair with a woman. There had been occasional visits from Franny, who would follow me anywhere, and the occasional meaningless orgy or threesome; but these were no more than fun, with little emotional involvement. This was different.

Of all the experiences I shared with Mathilde, the one that most transported me was when she bathed me. Once more I was the little girl in the tub: my mind flashed back to the way my mom would wash me from head to toe, soaping each of my feet as I held them in the air. My left foot she called "Sweet Johnnie," but since I always gave her a playful struggle over my right foot, it was nicknamed "Naughty Pete." He made her drop the soap and wet her blouse as she bent over to retrieve it. And I was delighted when her neatly combed hair got a bit disordered, especially when she washed my hair.

I recalled too the times on vacation when my mother and I showered together. Standing behind me, she would rub my back and under my armpits; I relished the briskness of her massage, and my skin glowed from the roughness of the loofah she used. But best of all were the sessions when she allowed me to rub down her own gorgeously firm body. I adored rubbing the thick, foamy soap over her back and shoulders, and sliding my hands down toward her buttocks. She never turned her front toward me to be washed, but I imagined it many times. The moment my dad came in and saw us together, she would find some excuse to shoo him off, or put an end to our little ritual, wrapping me in a huge bath towel and drying me off.

As Mathilde bathed me, I became that little girl once more. Leaning forward, she lingered lovingly over my arms before washing my hands, caressing each finger slowly and sensuously. Then she moved down to my thighs, brushing them briskly until my suntanned flesh glowed rosy red. I have shared many pleasurable baths with male lovers, but their hands never touched me in the way Mathilde did. I raised each foot for her attention, privately recalling "Sweet Johnnie" and "Naughty Pete" in my mind. Then she undressed and joined me in the tub, and it was my turn to anoint her sweet soft skin with lather. Unlike Germaine, Mathilde allowed me to soap and caress her front and back. Her body was smooth

and almost hairless, and I reveled in exploring its roundness and
the gentle swelling of her breasts. I gently soaped her pubic area
and tenderly parted the lips of her vagina, and as I placed a wisp of
foam inside she closed her eyes and moaned softly.

She washed and shampooed my hair; then, after she had blown
it dry, she wrapped my body in a thick woolly towel and led me into
her bedroom. She laid me on her bed and told me simply to relax
and enjoy whatever I felt. The body lotion with which she massaged
me had the scent of fresh lily of the valley, uncannily the same as
Germaine's favorite perfume.

For the first time in my life I was with a woman who made love
to me—who did everything she could to give me pleasure, bringing
me to a series of shattering orgasms instead of leaving me to serve
her passive needs.

Yet my ecstasy was mingled with a dreamlike confusion. With
my eyes closed, it was as though my lover were a creature of fantasy, a combination of myself in a few years to come, my mother a
few years ago, and Mathilde herself, here and now. What a rare,
heady experience, to be so pampered and mothered at the same
time! Mathilde, of course, was very much her own woman, no mere
shadow of any other. Yet to me our love affair evoked an unconscious desire I could never have admitted: to make love to my own
mother.

AFTERWARD, as I looked more closely at the objets d'art in her
living room, I discovered that Mathilde herself was a talented artist.
There were bottles transformed into gilded vases, each containing
a single bloom; tiny boxes became precious caskets, like richly
ornamented Russian jewel cases. And I fell in love with a gold-
painted candlestick she had created.

"Have you been painting long?" I asked.

"No, I only started about ten years ago. But ever since I was a child I wanted to be an artist. I spent all those years singing on those cruises; painting was just a hobby. It's only now that I truly have the time to make it my passion."

And this was perhaps the most surprising discovery of all. For my mother too had enjoyed just such a late-in-life conversion. When I was a child, of course, Germaine had been indifferent, even hostile, to Mick's artistic obsession. But later, when she was seventy, Hetty introduced her to a professional painter who also gave art classes. Under his guidance, she blossomed into an accomplished and passionate painter. I had found so many of Germaine's ways and tastes echoed in Mathilde; now, as I gaze at some of Germaine's own brightly colored canvases, it is my mother who brings back memories of my lover.

26

Living Together Apart

WITH JOHN living with me in Marbella, life was tempestuous. We were both used to having our own way, and though I never repeated my knife-throwing act, when we quarreled a hurricane of words flew between us. Such storms waned as suddenly as they arose, but my mother was often upset to see me subjected to abuse—yet, paradoxically, she remained genuinely fond of John even at the worst of times. He has done many things in his time, from dealing in high-performance cars to making movies, but in his youth he went straight from public school to art college and remains a dedicated and competent painter. So when Germaine started to paint, he appreciated her efforts and encouraged her, and their shared form of creativity created a bond between them.

The artistic link I shared with John was writing. While I persevered with my *Penthouse* column, he built a faithful following for a series of savagely satirical articles he wrote for *The Reporter*, a monthly tourist magazine published in Fuengirola. His comments on the Spanish social scene, on loutish tourists (usually English), and on feminist foibles were greeted with enthusiasm by the public. When I need a touch of brimstone in something I'm writing, and John is around, I can bypass the thesaurus: he's always there to help me express my anger. Being highly emotional as we both are is wonderful in bed, but less satisfying at the breakfast table: for years I've insisted on a simple breakfast of fresh orange juice in the morning, but my opponent persists in creating his expertly produced, high-cholesterol fry-ups. After shouting at him over his unwholesome diet, I inevitably make peace by helping him eat it: he's done wonders for my intellect but played havoc with my waistline.

Once, when we were alone and he was in a reasonable frame of mind, I opened my heart to him about our relationship—and about the touchy subject of infidelity, which was beginning to trouble me. "I don't care if you have ten different women once," I said, "but one woman ten times I can't accept. That way you give away your soul as well as your sperm. What would make me more than jealous—the one most hurtful and humiliating thing you could do to me—would be to share with someone else the little things we have in common. You know, our rituals—the silly things we say or do with each other and no one else. Treat some newfound lay like that, and *then* you'll hurt me."

"And you say you're not jealous?" he teased.

I remembered my father and his "banana skins," and how furious each relapse made Germaine. When she got over her feelings of betrayal she always knew that no one could undermine the foundation of her husband's love for her, but that didn't save her from outbursts of jealous rage. I could learn from her experience, and as far as I was concerned, John could break his neck on a whole street of banana skins, but when he brought his fancy bits of fruit home with him some accommodation had to be found if we were to remain living together.

AND IT WAS my mother who suggested the solution. Returning from a trip, I received an astronomical phone bill: John had been hosting some Canadian bird while I was away, and now it seemed I was being asked to finance the entire transatlantic cable. But Germaine urged me not to force a break with John over something as trivial as a phone bill.

"It's not just the money," I complained. "If John's going to keep bringing other women into this house, he'll leave me no space of my own. It's a big enough villa, for God's sake, but every time I come back from a trip I have to fight my way back into my own home. I feel like I'm suffocating."

"Then why don't you tell John you want the two of them to have their own quarters, and keep to them? Maybe he could use his own private space as well, and that way he can deal with her separately, without having to bother you."

Peace was restored. I paid to have a fully equipped kitchen installed in the guest wing of the villa: they would have their own living room and bedroom, in effect their own independent apartment. John was pleased to have his bedmate's fragile ego moved out of range of my tongue: I never resorted to blows, but she quaked in fear when I was on the warpath. After all, there was no point in destroying the life we'd spent twenty years building together for the sake of some trivial affairs. Now we could meet on the patio or in the garden, and we had our own space into which we could retreat. John even disconnected the speakers in my part of the house from the sound system I'd bought for him so that he could listen to his own classical music—day and night at full blast—while I enjoyed silence or my own music. The tension slackened, and something approaching harmony reigned: a kind of friendship even grew up between me and his girlfriend, who started to take my side in arguments when John's behavior was too outrageous. After a while, though, John simply grew bored with her, and she left.

So John and I live quite happily under one roof, and in what one of my friends once described as *casa caótica*, things have quieted down.

The way to live together, I had discovered, was sometimes to live apart.

BUT OUR TRANQUILLITY wasn't perfect. I did find a way to relax about money, after attending a weeklong consciousness-awareness course in Holland to overcome my suppressed anger and sense of powerlessness over the subject: when John called to ask me to send extra funds to cover various household expenses, I sent it without argument—no doubt disappointing him, as I'm sure he'd been storing up adrenaline for a fight. But soon we were arguing over other matters. He was frustrated by his failure to find a publisher for a book of his own, while I continued to be published, having built up relationships over many years. And when he vented his bitterness on me, I became so emotionally drained that I developed a writer's block of my own. I needed to find a man without John's assertiveness to bring some warmth back into my life, and although John had assumed the role of the dominant partner in Spain, in Amsterdam I came into my own.

The Café Scheltema is more than just a pub: it's a veritable institution. Authors, journalists, and all manner of creative artists congregate there, their conversation enlivened by the alchemy of wit and alcohol. At the back of the place, dominating the scene, is a large round marble table known to the regulars as the King's Table, in honor of the many celebrated Dutch writers whose initials had been chiseled into the stone there. It was understood that anyone so distinguished had thus claimed his place at the table for life.

I'd become something of a fixture at the table, and one evening, seeing the place of honor unoccupied, I installed myself at its head. Shortly thereafter, a photographer I'd known since my schooldays staggered in. No longer the attractive youth of old, he had degenerated into an abusive failure, and I wasn't thrilled when he flopped into a chair beside me and lit up a cheap, malodorous cigar. Pointing to his initials, he swore at me and ordered me out of "his seat." He probably took me for some submissive little girl, but parrying John's gibes and insults had hardened me up, and I think I bested him in the wrangle that followed. But the incident had soured the evening, and I decided to leave.

A firm believer in sexual equality, I had no hesitation in pushing my way into the men's rest room when I found the solitary women's washroom was occupied. I must have been more brusque than usual, for when I emerged a young man touched my arm.

"You know, you nearly crushed me against the wall as you rushed into the toilet," he said with a shy smile.

"So what? You survived, didn't you? What are you complaining about?"

I was still annoyed by my tussle with the drunken poetaster, but my anger abated as I took in the features of the youth I was arguing with now: his innocent blue eyes and slightly disheveled honey-colored hair were disarming.

"Well, what's your name?" I demanded.

"Romke. It's Romany," he added diffidently.

"You don't *look* very much like a Gypsy. I'd have guessed some Friesian village—a real Dutch cheese! And what's your claim to fame?"

"I'm a carpenter," he mumbled.

"Just what I need! Give me your phone number."

He fumbled for a pen, and I handed him one from the enormous bag I always lug around. He scribbled it on a coaster; I stuffed it in my bag and strode out to my car. And that was the start of a loving relationship that has lasted for six years.

A few days later, Romke and I started getting acquainted. He was working at a hospital as an apprentice carpenter and had to get to work at five every morning. But he spent most of his free time in my house, fixing scores of little things that had gone neglected for

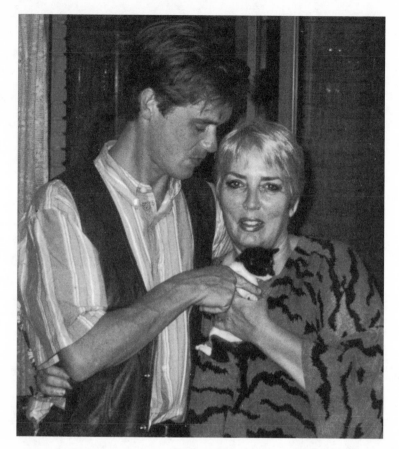

With Romke

years. He was very capable around the house—and, after a short course from me, also in bed. But I was a night owl: what use was a lover who was so exhausted by his day's work that he fell asleep at ten? Something had to give, and Romke gave up the drudgery of his daytime job and devoted all his time and energy to looking after me. When I brought him to Marbella, he was the perfect counterbalance to John. Soft-spoken and submissive, he was totally unmotivated by ambition. If John could take pride in having a girlfriend eighteen years his junior, I had the satisfaction of introducing my boyfriend, twenty-two years younger than I. And John found Romke's unassuming nature and obvious inexperience a welcome contrast to some of the frankly unsavory characters I turned to for company when things were at their worst between us.

GERMAINE'S REACTION, though, was another story. Romke was kind and faithful; he did my shopping, helped with the cooking, and generally acted as my right-hand man, always without complaint. Why couldn't she see how good we were together, how much he relieved me from the incessant fracas with John? It took Hetty to point out how much Germaine and Romke had in common. Both had moments of apparent aloofness when they couldn't bear being hugged or even touched by anybody; each was slow to open up to new acquaintances. But once they'd extended their trust to someone, both were fanatically loyal.

Maybe it was these very similarities that caused Germaine to keep her distance, but eventually she thawed and began to appreciate him. I took Romke with me to concerts and ballet, theater and film festivals, and we shared a taste for the macabre. After we'd been dating for a few months I persuaded him to sublet his own apartment and move in with me, which gave him some independent income. He was a free man, without any commitments, so we were able to travel the world together. I loved to spoil him mercilessly, and he was too shy to object, though he could become uncomfortable when my behavior became extravagant.

But most of the moments we shared were wonderful. Once, when we were in Venezuela, I hired a twin-engine plane to explore the magnificent waterfalls from on high. Romke was sitting in front of me, and I leaned against his shoulder as we gazed down at the brilliant colors of the landscape, the majestic mountain peaks and raging torrent beneath.

"Oh, Xaviera," he breathed. "That's amazing—it's *breathtaking!*"

There was no artifice to him: his simple unaffectedness was completely endearing. He was utterly without conceit—a refreshing contrast to John's worldliness. Not that I always gave him an easy time: deep down, he suffered from real insecurity, and whenever I lost my temper and shouted at him, he would retreat within himself in sulky silence or bury his nose in a book. Unlike John, he never retaliated in kind; indeed, I feel he loved me in part for the very dominance of my character. And when the occasion demanded, he could come up with a withering put-down. Once, at a party, I watched in amusement as an offensively drunken woman probably hoping to escape from her even more offensively drunken husband tried making a pass at him.

"Hey, kiddo," she called. "How old are you?"

"Twenty-four," Romke replied. "And you?"

"Thirty-five. Sorry, but you're too old for me," she teased.

"No, I'm sorry. You're too young for me," he retorted. "I like my women a little more . . . mature. Good-bye." He stood up and took me by the hand. "Let's get the hell out of here."

Fun indeed. But it would be in the days of my greatest distress that Romke proved his steadfastness and worth.

27

Life With
and Without Romke

ROMKE WAS A KIND and attentive companion, always deeply grateful for anything I did for him. But he did have problems that at times threatened our relationship. He'd come from a difficult background: there was a history of mental instability in his family, and Romke's life was a constant struggle against depression.

He tried periodically to find relief in drugs and drink, unaware that they actually aggravated his condition. My own tumultuous lifestyle simply overwhelmed him, and to calm his nerves he turned to drink and then to cocaine, and eventually began freebasing. He was mixing with the wrong sort of people—not just dealers but anyone with a sad story, some of whom he even allowed to stay in the basement of my house when I was in Spain. His behavior became erratic and aggressive, and this drove us apart. I have no patience with losers, which is what I thought he had become.

After Romke sublet his apartment, there was a crisis: eventually he found living under my roof too great a strain, but his tenant

refused to move, and the police refused to eject him. Virtually
thrown out of his own home and unwilling to return to mine, he
wandered the streets for half a year, often sleeping in the open. He
refused to lay off drugs himself, and refused to accept professional
help. I grew worried that in a fit of madness he might throw himself under a tram.

Yet it was Germaine, of all people, who managed to give him
back his self-confidence and peace of mind. Romke still had a key
to my house, and one day Germaine arrived to find him completely
out of control—literally foaming at the mouth. This was no new
experience for her—she must have seen Mick treating mentally dis-
turbed patients countless times—and by sheer force of her personality she persuaded him to sit quietly and unburden himself as she
listened with all the patience in the world. Calm was restored, and
before too long they were sipping a glass of sherry together.

This was the beginning of his rehabilitation. Germaine became
something of a substitute for Romke's mother, who lived far away
and had never been able to maintain any kind of helpful connection
with him. Germaine saw that Romke was basically a good kid, and
she was at pains to defend him to any casual visitors who dispar-
aged him or were frightened of him. With her help he managed to
kick his cocaine habit and moderate his drinking—which helped
him make a more convincing case to the police, who finally started
taking his complaints seriously and threw the squatter out of his
apartment. Then he barricaded himself inside his apartment until
he was clean.

Finally, Romke decided to give up trying to make a proper living taking odd carpentry jobs. Instead he took up social work as an
assistant nurse caring for the old and infirm—particularly those
who suffered from diseases like Alzheimer's—a job for which his
gentle character suited him well. And so, when Germaine herself at
last began growing ill, the kindnesses she had showed him were
repaid in kind.

ROMKE WASN'T the only one who was neglecting his body. I was going through a period of great strain, looking after my mom while trying to run a number of business ventures at the same time. I ignored my aches and pains, and put off long-overdue checkups until it was too late. Only when I was in sheer agony did I drag myself off to the gynecologist—and before I knew what was happening, I was rushed off to the hospital to undergo a complete hysterectomy.

I hadn't had any time to make the proper arrangements for a hospital stay, but when I called Romke and suggested he take over, he didn't hesitate for a moment. Our intimate relationship had broken off during his ordeal, but his feelings for me had never waned, and when I emerged from the hospital he was there to tend to me. We both had an unspoken desire to get back together, but Romke wasn't ready to make the first move; so for six weeks he looked after me and ran the house, even organizing a dinner party where my friends were seated around the hospital bed we'd set up in my living room. "We've finally got her where we want her," one of my friends said. "No more running off to some meeting—now she *has* to stay and listen to our stories."

Once I was given a clean bill of health, Romke moved back to his place to get on with his own life. I hired a live-in Californian cook, and from then on I was well cared for, at least around the house. But I also yearned for the love only another woman could provide.

In April 1997 I met Dia, a forty-five-year-old poet well known in the more intellectual lesbian circuit at the Cor Meyer, an old brown café in the heart of Amsterdam where once a month poets of different nationalities gather to read from their work.

Dia, whose body resembles mine when I was her age—round, feminine, and firm—had a very boyish quality, and I can't remember seeing her in a dress more than three times a year. Her dark

brown hair, cropped very short, gives her a definite look of androg-
yny. A champion swimmer with many a medal to her name, she
delighted in challenging other swimmers—not just for her own
gratification, but also to impress me. During the Gay Games in
Amsterdam she proudly presented me with several of her awards,
and eventually she found her own niche in my house to display
them, fastening on a little picture of herself in her black bathing
suit. I recognized the symptoms: Dia was just like me in my youth,
trying desperately to impress my father and earn his approval. Our
relationship was intense from the start: soon I realized I was more
than just a lover to her—I was also mother, sister, and friend.

Orphaned about ten years before we met, Dia was in a very real
way still grieving for her parents, and she often burst into spontaneous crying fits for no apparent reason. When I asked whether
she'd ever seen a psychiatrist, she said she'd been on Prozac for
years, but it hadn't really helped—and worse, it made it difficult for
her to reach orgasm. I convinced her to stop taking it, and her
depressions disappeared—replaced, happily, with a prodigious sexual appetite.

It was wonderful to be with a woman again—a soft, protective
force who wasn't afraid to show her emotions, her affection, her
need for love. Ours was the first real lesbian affair I'd had in years,
though I told her from the start that I was honestly bisexual, and
that Romke was still very much a part of my life. When I was
younger—until roughly my forties—men were the main objects of
my sexual interest, with lesbian lovers loitering in the background.
In my Happy Hooker days women were afraid I would seduce their
husbands away from them. Now it's the other way round: men are
my second choice, and the husbands get turned on by the prospect
of my seducing their wives.

Dia suffered anguish over my flirtations and occasional short
affairs with men. But she was utterly in love with me. Even now I
still feel awkward at her being so openly romantic: men like Romke,
Felix, even John, weren't given to such forthright pronouncements

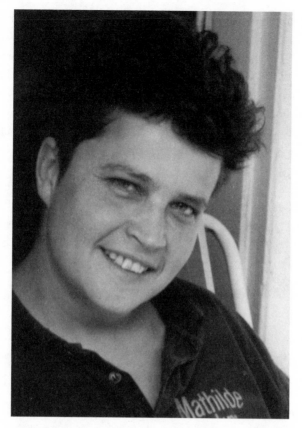

Dia

of devotion. But Dia was like a puppy, affectionate and obedient, and eager to help with the various projects in which I was always involved. Soon I found that she was helping bring order to my chaotic life—sorting out my business affairs, filing papers, devoting enormous attention to me whether I was being nice or nasty to her. She put up with my mood swings, though her pretty face would cloud over and her eyes grow wet with tears whenever I snapped at her, and she was also insanely jealous—aspects of our relationship I found difficult to accept.

Still, there's a lighter side to her character, and to our relationship. We both find great fun in zipping around town on my scooter, laughing our heads off, or dashing off to a department store in search of something as trivial as a new shower cap—not the kind of adventure likely to entertain a male companion. Our motto is, You need a good half dozen laughs to make a day worthwhile.

To this day Dia remains my lover and part-time housemate, and a delicate balance exists between her and Romke. Neither of them was ready to share my heart and my bed in the same house, so Romke amiably went back to his own apartment; once more he has his independence, though we're still the best of friends and occasional lovers, and neither he nor Dia harbor any real jealousy. Even my holidays are split among Dia, Romke, and John: though they occupy separate spheres of my life, they are my Three Musketeers, without whom I would be unable to exist.

NOW ROMKE is thirty-five years old, but he still has the same lean, strong body of the young boy I met eleven years ago. Not only has he given up booze and coke—he's even stopped smoking, whether cigarettes or grass. His sole indulgence is one fat, expensive cigar a day, and he's become quite the connoisseur. And as far as sex is concerned, there seem to be no other women in his life. From time to time a porno film might help him relieve his sexual tension, but the two of us still get together for the night about once a month, and when that happens it's a true feast.

28

From Cooker to Booker

IN 1980 I met Vaclav Vitvar, a Czech dissident who was introduced to me by the owner of one of Amsterdam's smaller English-speaking theaters. In their youth, Vaclav—who could have passed for Vladimir Lenin's twin brother—and his rosy-checked wife, Nora, had the art lovers of Prague at their feet with their cabaret act. One of the most widely read men I've ever met, Vaclav was also a fine musician, a pianist, organist, and composer who was liable to break into a spontaneous song-and-dance routine in the midst of a dinner party. And with Uncle Julius joining in with his cello, Vaclav spent hours at the keyboard in my Amsterdam home, their little ad hoc group entertaining us with every kind of music—from classical to Gypsy folk melodies, naughty ditties to Vaclav's original compositions.

Having quickly mastered the Dutch language, Vaclav and Nora were starting to build a new career in Amsterdam when Nora, barely fifty-five, developed cancer and died a short time later. Devastated, Vaclav moved to Germany, where he was offered a steady job as the organist at a Catholic church in Oberhausen.

But for me a flame had been lit, and from then on I made a practice of enlivening dinner parties with live music. Gradually over the
years I attracted a regular gathering of some of the city's finest
artists, men and women eager to talk and perform into the early
hours of the morning. My life had long since become too frantic for
housekeeping, so at the same time I hired a handful of excellent
cooks, whose efforts were greatly appreciated by my guests. I made
a special deal with most of them: free room and board, in exchange
for preparing three meals a day for me and a few guests. (Extra
guests, of course, meant extra pay.)

One of these cooks, a seasoned traveler named Steve who could
whip up a fabulous meal from just about any part of the world, suggested I start a kind of table d'hôte event in my house on a weekly
basis. For a set price, I provided a first-class, four-course meal, and
a bottle of wine. Each week there was a different theme: Mexican,
Indian, even Chinese, with a few Asian friends transforming the
room into a mock pagoda. On another occasion an Indonesian
rÿsttafel was served by waiters in sarongs, with appropriate music.
The food Steve prepared was delicious and looked sensational.
Soon the event began turning into a genuine singles scene, and at
least every other week I brought in a musician or actor to perform
during the meal. For the growing number of guests, these evenings
offered a cozy night on the town in a homey restaurant—much
more than simple food and drink.

The climax of these "Happy Cooker" evenings was undoubtedly Valentine's Day, when it seemed as if every romantic couple in
the city was making a beeline for my place. I'd been trying to limit
the numbers, but the house was jam-packed, and that night no less
than sixty sat down for dinner. Hot and cramped it may have been,
but it was so lively that everyone had a wonderful time. In the middle of the meal, some of the guests got up and started giving
impromptu performances on my piano and two guitars; two
women grabbed the mikes and started belting out "My Funny

Valentine," and a concert pianist sitting nearby sat in to provide professional accompaniment.

But now the time had come for a change—for a different artistic direction, you might say.

Since 1980 I'd been attending the Edinburgh International Festival, sampling from among literally thousands of shows; my old friend David lived in that city now and helped me choose promising events while guiding me through the labyrinthine city to help me avoid traffic. Sometimes John accompanied me, and we made a great team, on occasion attending up to four performances a day. For once we were totally on the same wavelength and would take a break for a day or two to see something of the spectacularly beautiful countryside.

It was during these yearly trips that I got hooked on the theater. We enjoyed everything, from comedy acts like Earl Okin, who became a friend, to the Liverpool poet Roger McGough, a particular favorite of John's. We especially relished the mind-blowing solo performances and full-length plays of Steve Berkoff, a fascinating writer/director/actor I first met in Sydney, long before he achieved fame with a macabre stage adaptation of Kafka's *Metamorphosis*.

Suddenly I knew what my life's ambition had always been: to find a way to share such brilliant performances with my friends in Holland. I resolved to bring to Amsterdam the best from Edinburgh and beyond.

WITH THE ESTABLISHMENT of my own theater, Xaviera's Theatre Restaurant, I outgrew the Happy Hooker image at last and fought my way into the respectable world of the arts. I believe Mick would have been proud.

Early on, I made the decision that my theater would concentrate on English-language performance—a decision that provoked some commentary in the press. But the fact is that right now there is no other English-language theater in the whole of Holland, apart from a few stand-up comedy venues—yet there is a significant English-speaking population living and working in the Amsterdam area, craving for entertainment in their own language. I would present outstanding Dutch artists as well, but the tourists and expats from Australia, America, England, Ireland, and South Africa would be my core audience.

And what good fortune: my home was a natural venue. I could seat fifty diners—space enough for a reasonable-size audience. Together with a few friends, Romke transformed one end of my long living room into a stage. My furniture safely stored away, I bought seventy comfortable velour folding chairs, and made a deal with a light-and-sound technician friend who allowed us to store his equipment in my garden shed in exchange for letting us use it whenever we needed. As the track lighting and blackout curtains fell into place, so did the team I needed to make the project, work—among them James, who'd been my gardener in Spain but moved to Amsterdam to serve as my general factotum, and Chris, a sensitive gay Asian photographer who lives in and keeps the place immaculate. Now, in addition to looking after me, the two of them took on a new key function: providing catering services for my audiences. Along with a dozen young energetic helpers recruited to design and distribute flyers and press releases and maintain a marketing database, this is what I call the X Team: my virtual family, who have made the venture a success.

THOUGH I WAS still scouting for English-language productions, Xaviera's Theatre Restaurant actually opened in fall 1996 with an autobiographical play by the actress Sylvia de Leur, a friend and contemporary of mine. Sylvia's mother was Czech, her father a Dutch Jew; her account of her childhood infatuation with her father, to the distress of her mother, obviously struck a chord with me. And the guest of honor at the opening was none other than my own mother.

Germaine looked radiant, her hair coiffed to perfection, her makeup beautiful. She wore an elegant black dress with white dots, and a matching scarf round her neck in that style I could never imitate. Hetty came in a black and red pantsuit and sat where my mom told her, and shortly afterward they were joined by Romke's mother. While Hetty was busy inspecting the kitchen, Romke surreptitiously slipped a whisky to his mother and a sherry to mine. In fact, Hetty was so busy nosing around that they managed to get in a second round before Hetty returned to join them near curtain time.

It was lovely to see the two mothers get along so well, as the two of them slowly grew tipsy together. Germaine became quite emotional by the end of the play; she had known Sylvia since my teenage years, and now here she was—mature, rounder, sharing her warmest emotions for her mother, who had recently passed away. As a child, Sylvia had suffered: her mother was tyrannical and sank into alcoholism. Yet every word Sylvia spoke shone with love for her mother, despite all the pain she had endured. Love, forgiveness, and compassion were her subjects, and many in her audience were moved to tears.

I had a full house, and word of mouth ensured the same in the days to come. Both the play and the house-theater concept itself got wonderful reviews. Some called me the Queen of Kitsch: my house was full of wooden masks from Bali, statues flown in from Mexico, marble masks from Uruguay, an entire collection of ceramic turtles and frogs, and my collection of novelty lighters and ashtrays. But everyone seemed charmed by the entertainment, the setting, and the clientele.

And faithfully, until shortly before her death, Germaine attended all my productions. As her neurotic daughter dashed around, calling her with news of the latest bookings or newspaper gossip, she remained calm as a ship in harbor.

At last, I felt, she had become proud of her daughter.

29

Whose House Is It?

IN AMSTERDAM, even as a lively theater raged within it—my house always was my undisputed territory. I could come and go as I pleased, invite my friends without having to suffer unwanted guests. In Spain, it was a different matter. John was now so firmly entrenched that at times I felt like no more than a tolerated guest in my own home. John even started to become impatient with my mother—and in particular with Hetty. Swallowing my resentment, I secured an apartment for them in town, where for years they spent six weeks or so each spring. In the end, it proved a convenience: they had no car in Spain, and my villa was too remote for Hetty to go out shopping early while my mom was still asleep.

Soon they'd begun making a life of their own in Marbella and found new friends. One was Jana, a bighearted Dutchwoman who'd enjoyed a full life before retiring to an apartment overlooking the beach. Before she met Germaine and Hetty, her existence had been largely housebound, but Germaine and Hetty were charmed by her, and I was comforted that they'd found someone to depend on when I wasn't around. Jana always had a big, happy smile for Germaine, and my mom found her such a warm, sympathetic friend that now and again she even called her from Holland when she needed cheering up.

One morning, Hetty had arranged to meet Jana for breakfast. This gave me a welcome opportunity to spend time alone with my mother, so I was there to wake her at ten with fresh croissants, hot coffee, and a copy of *De Telegraaf*. When I brought in the tray she was still sound asleep, so I slipped off my dress and snuggled into bed behind her. I put my arm around her shoulders and gently rubbed her neck. She stirred slightly, uttered some sleepy noises, and made one of her little hand gestures that meant *Keep quiet, I'm not quite ready to wake up*. She probably thought it was Hetty, giving her a good-morning cuddle.

Languidly, she turned to face me and opened her eyes.

"Ach, mein piekeltje," she gasped in amazement—a special term of endearment she used just for me, her charming German accent suddenly sneaking into her words. She took both my hands and kissed them. She must have been quite surprised, as I'd never snuck into bed with her anywhere outside Amsterdam. I was about to speak, but she put her finger on my lips and whispered to me to keep silent.

"Don't worry, I am awake," she assured me. "I just want to enjoy these unforgettable moments with my child. These are moments that no one can take away from me." We both seemed to sense that this might be a farewell to our lifelong ritual.

It had been a long time since we last had shared a bed together. I had almost forgotten how familiar her body felt, though it was much older now than when we last slept together. I will never forget the sweet smile on her face, her eyes half-closed, as she softly brushed her cheek against mine, how she coyly removed her pink hairnet as I planted a good-morning kiss on the tip of her nose and one on her forehead. Our fingers intertwined as we hugged each other, nestled in spoon fashion, inhaling each other's fragrances.

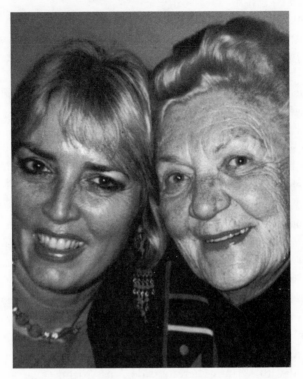

With Germaine, 1988

Sipping her coffee in bed, we talked about how much she still missed Mick's presence in her life, and how his death had affected her. And about what it was like living with Hetty, day in and day out.

I understood how she felt. She was a woman who would have liked to change her life drastically after the death of her husband but suddenly realized she was too old to do so. Years spent tending a sick husband, and another six living alone, had taken their toll: she had aged rapidly, and in her loneliness she had started to feel powerless. Unable to change her ways, she had become enslaved by Hetty, who loved nothing more than looking after her girlfriend and catering to her every whim—but at the same time controlling her life.

After her second cup of coffee and our long chat, I offered to help her up so we could continue breakfast in the living room. "My child," she whispered, "it's almost as if you have come home again from a long journey. Tell me, where has Hetty got to anyway?"

"Mom," I said, "I just felt like being a good daughter and spoiling you. Hetty is having breakfast with Jana; she won't be back for a while. Let's get you out of bed and dressed. We can have our croissants while they're still warm, and then drive into town if you like. Okay?"

She agreed eagerly; seldom had I seen her look so happy. I helped her get out of bed, and as she clasped my shoulders I gently led her into the bathroom. She asked me to run a bath for her— something she hadn't done for a very long time—so I mixed some bubbly foam in a warm bath. Then I helped her carefully out of her nightgown and into the rather low bathtub. I washed her shoulders and back, then left her for a while, since I knew how much she enjoyed simply soaking in the bubbles.

I made her bed and set about tidying up the kitchen, and must have lost track of time until I heard a faint cry for help and dashed into the bathroom. She had been lying there for some twenty minutes, unable to move and too embarrassed to call for me until she realized she had no choice.

"I can't seem to get out of this bathtub," she whined softly. "It is horrible to grow old and be so dependent. You know how much I've always loved taking baths."

Still naked myself, I leaned forward, took her gently by her thin arms, and lifted her bodily out of the bathtub. I had forgotten how fragile her bones were, and she moaned a little as she shifted her weight to me. I finally placed her on a bath mat in front of the sink and helped her towel herself dry. It struck me that some forty years had passed since I had last seen another woman her age—my father's mother, Grandma Esther—naked in the bathroom. She too had become stuck in the bathtub, and as her son helped her, I remember standing and watching in amazement.

Now Germaine stood before the mirror, applying cream to her face. Gazing over her shoulder into the mirror, I couldn't help noticing that her breasts, which I had adored and envied as a child, were still quite firm, though smaller than I remembered. But they still were in great shape, especially for a woman her age. Everything about her seemed somehow to have diminished in size, and there were a few rough patches on her once-smooth skin. I sat her on the toilet seat to massage her with baby oil I warmed in my hands, and gently kneaded her frail shoulders. Her skin was dry as parchment, but it seemed to come miraculously back to life. I had just finished when we heard the key in the front door. All at once Hetty was there, standing in the doorway, stupefied to see the two of us naked together.

"What the heck are you two doing here, if I may ask?" she demanded.

"I came to bring over some croissants, and then I decided to run a bath for Mom. I was just helping her out, rubbing some oil into her skin. Do you mind?"

I helped my mother up, and we made our way, arm in arm, to her bedroom so that she could choose some clothes for the day.

"Amazing!" Hetty exclaimed. "Do you know you two look exactly alike from the back? You have exactly the same buttocks and hips. Of course, Xaviera has more meat on her bum, but you even walk the same way. It's uncanny."

HETTY'S REACTION that morning was typical. Romke and I were usually exceptions, but she was extraordinarily possessive, harboring resentment for any visitors who might seem to threaten her dominion. In her later years Germaine sometimes felt lonely and isolated, but when she called old friends to pay her a visit, Hetty often found a way to scuttle the plan. One friend, a sweet, kindhearted woman named Mientje, adored Germaine and gladly made the two-hour trip to Amsterdam when she called—only to be turned away at the door by Hetty, with the excuse that Germaine wasn't well enough to see her. When I was in town, Germaine's calls to me to come and pick her up were often rushed, as if she were afraid of being caught on the phone. After Germaine's death I learned that Hetty often called to cancel such arrangements.

I once asked my mother why she sometimes seemed so timid on the phone. To my surprise, she told me that Hetty—always obsessed with cameras, videos, and gimmicks of every kind—had taken to taping her phone calls. Apparently Germaine had found out about it after calling me one day to complain about something—only to be reprimanded for it by Hetty after she'd returned and listened to the call.

"So that's why you're so paranoid about saying anything confidential when we talk," I said. "But can't you stop her? After all, it's your house and your phone, isn't it?"

My mom laughed sardonically. "Yes, my child—as much as your villa in Spain is yours. Doesn't John have just as vicious a grip over you when you're there?"

Understandably, Germaine found Hetty's wiretapping hobby a vexing invasion of her privacy. Yet I'm not sure she fully realized just how hooked Hetty was on her, and how much she enjoyed pleasing her in her own peculiar, almost submissive, way. My mother had only to snap her fingers and ask for a cup of coffee, a biscuit, her pills, or anything, and Hetty would dash to do her bidding. Hetty was crippled by rheumatism; at times every step was agony. But she would drive to the other end of town if Germaine suddenly took a fancy for a herring and chopped-onion sandwich, or fresh strawberries and cream in midwinter.

Although in Holland each kept her own place and had her own car, the two women were together day and night. Each needed the other: Germaine's presence gave Hetty dignity and a sense of self-worth, while Hetty offered Germaine company and literally kept her alive as old age slowly robbed her of her health. Their secret sign language was intricate and unmistakable: a finger to her mouth meant *Don't wake me up yet*, another, more vigorous wave of the hand meant *Open the curtain a bit*, and holding a phantom cup to her lips meant *It's time for coffee*. And when she moved her hand up and down twice, palm downward, it could mean *Take it easy, Don't rush me*, or *Turn down the music*. At the end of her life, when she grew too weak to speak, this sign language became a gift to me as well.

GERMAINE BECAME gradually more lethargic in her eighties, and often she did not react to my questions, only smiling sweetly. With her eyes fixed in a gentle stare, her wrinkled face seemed to soften, and she began to look younger and carefree. She was fond of saying that the eyes were the mirror of the soul, but now hers were often quite expressionless, and I could no longer see through them to what was going on in her mind. Sometimes she would snap out of her apathy and become alert and talkative, but more often when I asked her a question Hetty would break in and answer before Germaine had a chance to open her mouth. But eventually my words seemed to go in one ear and out the other. She hadn't grown senile, but she grew forgetful and unaware of day-to-day problems, as if she were living in a world of her own, and her face would assume an expression of childlike happiness.

For many years my mom had recorded all my income and expenses in a ledger that I termed my famous green book. This wasn't only for my benefit: it was also her way of keeping hold over me, making sure I would come visit her at least twice a week with a handbag full of bills that needed paying. She would write out all my checks and bank orders, enabling me to go traveling for as long as I wanted without worrying whether my bills were getting paid. But now it was clear I would need to start doing my own book-keeping, and I bought my own large book—red this time, but otherwise identical to the original. She reluctantly accepted the new arrangement; it was growing harder for her to cope with complicated matters, and her handwriting started to get a bit shaky. She had missed a few items of late; her lapses weren't of any real importance, but she'd always been proud of her memory, and they caused her great alarm. Now I began keeping the books myself, my higgledy-piggledy scrawl nestling together with her orderly Germanic figures. But Germaine insisted on supervising everything I did, and ordered me to keep both ledgers under her roof—for my protection, she said.

IN MARBELLA my mom decided each summer that one of her ailments must be treated by some new Dutch specialist she had found in the area. Treatment was quicker than in Holland, and half the price. Hetty loved to visit hospitals, although apart from her rheumatism she was rarely ill. But with Germaine hospitals and doctors were an obsession, almost certainly a leftover from her days as Frau Doctor de Vries: for years she had insisted on driving around in my dad's old car with its M.D. designation on the windshield—although this was strictly illegal and she was always at risk of being stopped to treat some accident victim.

Germaine and Hetty had a regular taxi driver who understood their passion for hospitals, and one day he pointed out the new Marbella Clinic, a sparkling white building still under construction. Germaine insisted on stopping to inspect the place, and when she discovered that the cafeteria was open, she decided it was the perfect place for lunch. When I heard this latest streak of morbidity, I flew into a rage.

"What is it with the two of you and this craze for hospitals? You're on vacation—why can't you eat in a normal restaurant?"

My mom shouted back, "It's *none of your business* what we do with our time."

In no time we were at it hammer and tongs, our fiercest row in many years. The only reason Germaine didn't throw me out of the house was that I stormed out first, slamming the door behind me.

"And don't come back. I don't want you to set foot in this flat ever again," she called after me.

I suppose she had the right to ban me from her apartment—though of course I paid for it. But the following week was hell for both of us. I couldn't sleep and developed migraine attacks. When I did close my eyes, the nightmares returned. As for Germaine, I learned later, she had become so tearful and moody that Hetty was preparing to book them an early flight home. Normally my mother and I couldn't bear being away from each other for more than a day or two when we were in the same city, but German pride and Dutch obstinacy are two powerful forces.

Every time my phone rang I ran to it, hoping in vain that it would be her. But one day something terrible happened: I picked up the phone, and the voice on the other end was that of Maria, an undertaker with a flourishing funeral business.

"Does your mother have a blue velvet coat and a pair of white pants?" she asked.

"Yes," I said in a panic. "Why do you want to know?"

"Well, I think we may have found her dead on the street in front of that hairdresser where she usually goes. Isn't that near where you used to live?"

I gasped for air. John was standing beside me. He grabbed the phone and asked Maria to repeat what she'd said.

John repeated her words to me: "A woman of your mother's age and appearance died of a heart attack, and was found on the street."

"Can I go to identify the body? For God's sake, where do I have to go?" I cried.

"She's in the morgue."

The morgue.

"She has another question," he said, handing me back the phone.

"Did she wear white high heels?" Maria asked.

I sighed with relief. My mother always wore special brown sandals, low and flat, to support her sore feet.

"That's good, then. Let me call you back in fifteen minutes."

The minutes until she called back were the longest I ever lived through. When she called again, it was to reassure me that the dead woman was someone else.

But the trauma was enough to send me dashing over to my mother's house. I got there to find them standing amid packed suitcases; we had a good cry, and as Hetty put away the big bunch of red roses I'd brought, I promised that we'd never leave each other on such bad terms again. I convinced them to change their tickets back, and we spent the next two blissful weeks together.

WHEN I STOPPED by one morning, two days before our departure, Hetty begged me to come to the bedroom where my mother was still half-asleep and feel her left breast. Apparently Germaine had noticed some lumps a few weeks before, but after our fight she had been shy about bothering me with her problems. Once again panic-stricken, I called a radiologist for an immediate appointment. The hours waiting for the results of the X rays were interminable.

When eventually we were summoned to his office, the expression on the doctor's face confirmed our fears. Two large X rays were hanging on the wall, and on one there was a chain of black dots. For an instant, I held out hope that they were from different patients, and the clear one was Germaine's. But they were pictures of both her breasts, one of which was cancerous.

Germaine was devastated but didn't shed a tear. Hetty was overwhelmed; she couldn't stop crying, and the doctor finally gave her a Valium to tranquilize her. I called Holland immediately and made an urgent appointment at van Leeuwen hoek Ziekenhuis, one of Holland's finest cancer hospitals. We flew to Amsterdam that night, and Germaine was in the hospital the following morning.

30

Germaine and Suffering

GERMAINE HAD BEEN WHEELED into the operating theater. Hetty and I waited, breathless with anxiety. There was nothing to do now but wait and then wait some more, hour after hour. We went to the coffee shop but were too fraught to swallow a drop of coffee or eat a crumb of bread. The coffee shop was just somewhere to go.

The first glimmer of hope came when a nurse told us the patient had been moved to the recovery room, adjacent to the operating theater. The operation had taken well over four hours, and we had been on tenterhooks every second. Germaine had been the oldest patient in the ward. Tough old biddy that she was, though, she made it.

We were allowed to go down to see her, though we were warned that she was still only semiconscious and we probably wouldn't be able to communicate with her.

Her face was swollen and reddish, and her eyes were closed. Bending over her, I could make out the words she was mumbling:

"Pain, pain. *Mutti, Mutti.*" It was something of a shock to me: just as I would call on my mother for comfort, here was my mother calling out for hers, long dead though she was.

There was nothing we could do; we simply stood there by her side, willing the pain to go away. After ten minutes the surgeon walked in, shook hands, and congratulated us.

"So what did you do?" I asked. "Did you have to remove her left breast?"

"No, madam." He came straight to the point. "I amputated both breasts. One was so heavily cancerous that I couldn't risk the cancer spreading to the other. So we performed a preventative operation. I hope you can accept this. Remember, she has reached a respectable age."

Her breasts, which just a few weeks earlier I had washed and dried so tenderly in the bath in Marbella. Her breasts, so proudly displayed when she was young, in a negligee or low-cut dress. But these were also the breasts that had dried up at the outbreak of the war, denying her milk to feed the beloved baby she had so desperately brought into the world.

A couple of hours later, after Hetty and I had eaten something, we were able to visit Germaine again, this time in her own room. An awful shock awaited us: a group of doctors surrounded her bed, working furiously. One explained to us that she'd suffered a relapse and her temperature had fallen sharply. They were shouting at her, slapping her face in a frantic effort to resuscitate her. All the ruddiness had left her cheeks, now gaunt and deathly pale; her hollow eyes stared, her teeth chattered. Hetty and I sat huddled in a corner, praying that the doctors could pull off a miracle. Half an hour passed before her breathing became normal and the icy fever subsided.

Hetty and I came each day and provided my mother with what comfort we could. She certainly didn't receive much from the nursing staff, who were far too busy to display much compassion. There was an exception, though, in one sweet-tempered nurse who always had time to exchange a few words with Germaine. She was in her midfifties, quite a bit older than the other nurses on the ward, and a bond of sympathy grew up between the two women.

One day I asked whether she didn't feel a bit lonely. "Not really," she replied. "I can usually take off a few minutes with my daughter."

"Does she work far from here?" Hetty asked.

"The other side of the corridor. She's an oncology nurse here too."

It seemed strange to me that they didn't work together; she explained that her daughter had volunteered to nurse children who had developed tumors, and she herself couldn't handle the strain of watching youngsters fading each day.

When Germaine started to feel a bit stronger, quite a few women on the ward would drop by her room to chat. Many of them took a liking to her; she became a kind of mother confidante, and though she was still weak, they brought her all of their social as well as medical problems.

Germaine certainly was brave; of the twenty-four women in the ward, she became one of the few who survived for some years. But after her operation, her entire lifestyle changed. She suddenly became an old woman and seemed to lose her appetite for life. A nurse now came every morning to bathe and dress her, but whenever she got a glimpse of her flat, scarred chest she would burst into tears. She threw away every mirror she could lay her hands on, and began to neglect her appearance. She had always worn makeup every day—immaculate lipstick and mascara—but now she only bothered if she had to leave the house.

All the fun seemed to go out of her life; she never picked up a paintbrush, choosing instead to flick listlessly through the pages of gossip magazines or sit in front of the television. The doctors had said it was vital that she keep moving, so she got herself a home trainer, and with the help of a massage at least three times a week, we managed to keep her pretty mobile. But the problem was more than physical: I wanted her to recapture her will to live, to stop talking about dying all the time.

Her pains seemed to get worse each day, and every time she sensed a new pain or discovered a lump in her body she hadn't noticed before, she was seized by panic. She would scream to Hetty to take her back to the hospital, convinced that the doctors had lied and her cancer had recurred. Ever obedient, Hetty would dress her in warm clothes, manhandle her out the door, and drive her to the nearest doctor or hospital, where Germaine would be examined and always declared cancer-free. The same pantomime occurred in Marbella, with myself or her sympathetic taxi driver taking over Hetty's role. Always the result was negative. But whenever she was upset—often about me—or under stress, her abdominal pains would erupt with renewed ferocity, leaving her medical consultants powerless to help.

But Germaine wasn't the only old lady suffering. Her rheumatism growing worse, Hetty was now taking half an hour to creep from her bed to the bathroom in the morning. Her condition was so severe that her doctor prescribed a week's stay in a specialized clinic; but she refused to go, unwilling to leave my mother alone. But if she was looking for a word of comfort or sympathy from her girlfriend, she was disappointed.

"Don't exaggerate! Your pains are nothing compared to mine. You've had that rheumatism as long as I've known you. I'm the one who's practically bedridden. You can manage on your own; all you're after is sympathy from me and my daughter."

Germaine clearly wasn't herself. But there came a time when Hetty couldn't put up with it any longer and announced she was going back to live in her own house.

Germaine grabbed the phone and called me. "Guess what? Hetty's leaving again. I'm sure it's all talk. She's crying her crocodile tears in the bedroom with the door closed, but she's probably got her ear against the door listening to us right now. She'd never dare leave me—she's never had it so good in her entire life."

She paused, waiting for me to comment. I kept my mouth shut. "I look after all her needs. There's no rent to be paid, no food bills to be taken care of. All she has to do is make me one meal a day, and a few cups of coffee. And you know what? She always boils her vegetables in the morning, and just heats them all up again at night. Do you call that healthy eating? There can't be a single vitamin left in that mess."

Another pause, but I kept silent, waiting for the storm to blow itself out. "Ugh . . . I cannot *stand* the food she prepares for me, nine times out of ten. I don't know if you know it, Vera, but she never seems to wash her hands before she starts cooking. I find that disgusting. Maybe it's best if she leaves after all. I can look after myself."

I heard her yell, "Hetty, why don't you go, then, and leave me alone? I don't ever want to see that ugly face of yours again."

"So, Mom, what do you think you'll do without Hetty?" I asked when she turned back to the phone.

"Don't you worry. I can manage on my own, thank you," she said sourly.

That was nonsense; there was no way she could look after herself. She relied on a nurse to wash and dress her, and she couldn't even go to the bathroom without assistance. She had not been out shopping for at least a year, and whatever she might say about Hetty's cooking, she hadn't made herself so much as a cup of coffee for months.

At the moment, it turned out, Hetty was just bluffing. But soon I became really alarmed: what would happen if Hetty ever did leave? I knew it would be impossible for my mom to move in with me; she could never cope with the incessant stream of visitors or guests, the hubbub of my normal life. I suggested very tentatively that we might consider the prospect of a retirement home. Waiting lists could be as long as four years, and the costs horrendous, but some places were comfortable houses standing in their own gardens, with what amounted to a separate apartment for each resident. I was able to persuade the two old ladies to come and inspect one such home, conveniently close to my house so that I could make weekly visits; I told them it was really just a kind of hospital, hoping to appeal to their morbid side.

As we drove up, the sight of the porter in his cubbyhole at the gateway seemed to awaken a memory for Germaine. In her confused state of mind she was suddenly back in Indonesia, confronted by a prison guard; she flew into a panic, and it was ten minutes before she was calm enough for us to go inside.

As it happened, the residents weren't so much gray panthers as blue-rinse doves. As we sipped weak tea, charming young male nurses cosseted them while they swapped the latest gossip and inquired whether "darling" or "sweetie" had slept well.

But many of the permanently waved women and bald old men, hobbling painfully along with the aid of a cane or walker, were pitiably frail, and my mother found very little tempting about the prospect of sharing living quarters with them. At another facility we visited, the inmates immediately brought to mind the poor people my father used to treat from the working-class district of Amsterdam: simple, straightforward men and women, plain folks with no pretense of sophistication—and definitely not the sort of people with whom Germaine had a lot in common.

She did ultimately consent to go on a waiting list, and after six months we were phoned with the news that there was an apartment available. But then Germaine went berserk, screaming that the only way she'd ever leave her own home would be "horizontal, in my coffin." Her name was removed from the list.

That evening I had a serious talk with Germaine and told her she'd better change her tune with Hetty and start behaving reasonably, or she might really move out. Then we'd have to find another nurse, who would help put Germaine to bed and give her meals, but that would be all. She would be left on her own for the rest of the day and night. And if she ever misbehaved toward a nurse the way she tormented poor Hetty—whether at home or in an

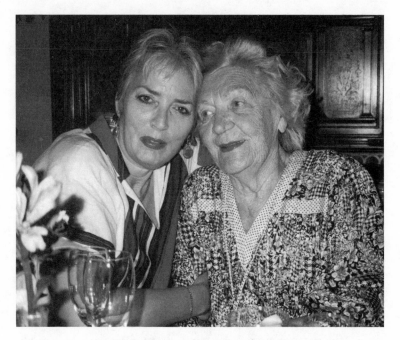

Around the time of Germaine's operation

institution—the nurse would probably leave her to lie in her own piss. Germaine must have been listening; the following day she had calmed down considerably and called a truce with her companion, grumbling like a small child whose toys had been taken away.

To be fair, I had a lot of sympathy for my mother; my own hysterectomy had affected me emotionally, and for Germaine the double mastectomy must have been worse yet. And with the quality of her life dwindling so dramatically, she must have felt her life coming to an end.

WHEN SHE WAS EIGHTY-THREE her stomach pains got worse, and she insisted that Hetty put the hottest of hot water bottles on her bare stomach. She refused to have it inside a wool sleeve, and when Hetty did slip it inside a towel, Germaine would surreptitiously remove it. After a few months her skin was a network of blue blotches and brown scorch marks, a sad contrast to the pure white smooth flesh I remembered holding as a child or massaging with suntan oil on the Côte d'Azur.

Despite her self-neglect, until the end of her life my mother maintained her shapely, graceful hands, and I delighted in giving her a manicure. She had the strongest nails I've ever encountered, and when she was going out or expecting visitors, I would change her nail polish from her customary fiery red to a gentler shade of pink and persuade her to put on a softer lipstick. I still took every opportunity to soothe her fragile skin with baby oil, and gave the same loving treatment to her feet, enjoying the sensation of her dead skin coming back to life under my fingers.

At such times my mom was docile and uncomplaining, but she wasn't always in a mellow mood. As is common with former cancer patients, she had fits of crying, but above all she suffered from a fear of senility, and her feelings of powerlessness were certainly at the root of her problems with Hetty.

And she showed a dogged determination to defend her independence until late in life. When she was seventy-eight, pulling out of a gasoline station, she accelerated onto the highway far too slowly and was hit by a Porsche that totaled her car. Miraculously, neither woman was hurt, thanks to the seat belts they wore. There was no doubt that Germaine was at fault, so when she rebuked a young police officer who spoke to her less than respectfully, she lost her driver's license. When she pleaded with me to get it restored, I explained that getting a new license would mean attending a driving school, taking a so-called refresher course as though she were a new driver, and then passing a stringent test at the end. That, I thought, was the end of that.

To my amazement and that of all our friends, a few months later she waved a trophy before my eyes: a new license. She had persevered with the course and passed the test with flying colors.

"You're kidding! Let me see that!" I asked, reaching for the card. But she just kept waving it playfully above her head, safely out of my reach. In fact, Germaine never allowed anyone to see her driver's license or her passport, as she altered her date of birth to suit her mood, and would never admit to her true age. I knew her birthday was May 2, but sometimes the year was 1914, sometimes 1916; when she was really in top form she was known to reach for 1918.

These petty fibs became absolutely silly when she was in her late seventies. She still looked great; what was the point in knocking ten or fifteen years off her age, as if she were her own long-lost younger sister? I tried to point out the downside of her strategy—instead of admiring her for being so well preserved in her seventies, they'd just think she was an especially wrinkled sixty-year-old—but this always led to a furious row.

And there were other bones of contention. I had a habit of turning down the central heating as soon as I entered their apartment; the temperature was stifling, and it never occurred to me that old people might feel the cold more intensely. I would sometimes even open a window to let in a blast of fresh air. When they knew I was coming, they would turn down the heat themselves, like a couple of naughty kids afraid of being caught by the stern headmistress. Of course, the moment my back was turned, up would go the heat again.

I also scolded my mother about her diet. "Why am I always catching you eating white bread and jam instead of a good healthy salad? You need plenty of vitamins, like in fresh orange juice. At least get Hetty to buy whole wheat bread instead of that plastic rubbish."

That was the last straw. Her face grew red, and she gave as good as she got. "Who are you to preach to me about my diet? There was a plate of sweets on that table when you came in. Where are they now? You gobbled every single one. If you live to be as old as I am, I hope you'll be as fit as I am, but if you keep stuffing yourself, you won't live that long! So mind your own business and stop inter-fering all the time."

She was absolutely right, but it was still a slap in the face.

BUT GERMAINE'S twilight years weren't all unrelieved misery. We did our best to bring back a little sunshine into her life. Both Hetty and Germaine enjoyed birthday celebrations, but the great event was Christmas. I used to throw big parties in my house, but after Germaine turned eighty she preferred a quieter, more intimate setting in her own apartment. So Romke and I arrived, each bear-ing gifts, mine something very special. Hetty welcomed us at the door with a hush and handed Romke a Santa Claus costume to put on in the bedroom. He emerged trailing a long white beard, sport-ing the traditional red hat and Hetty's father's pince-nez perched on the tip of his nose. He quite took Germaine by surprise, dis-pensing gift-wrapped packages from a large basket and wishing her a happy Christmas in a deep, melodious voice while planting a kiss on her cheek.

Hetty had come into her own. Taking out my mom's best Wedgwood chinaware, she spread before us neatly decorated plates of snacks and drinks. The room was festooned with dozens of cards, and fairy lights were strung around photographs of my par-ents and me. Candles flickered in front of a collage she made from photographs of some of Germaine's paintings. Every year Hetty had a lovely calendar made of these photographs as a kind of Christmas gift to send to friends all over the world.

I'd warned Hetty that my present might evoke emotional mem-ories for Germaine, and at the appropriate moment she made sure to hand Santa the video recorder. After a lot of effort I had man-aged to find a video of the prologue to *Pagliacci*, and as the golden voice of Placido Domingo rang through the room, my mom's eyes filled with tears. How often, when she felt depressed or misunderstood by her husband, had she found solace in Caruso's famous rendition, when I was barely a teenager and she still a gorgeous young woman.

We sat, huddled together, watching the bitter tears of the clown as he put on the greasepaint, heartbroken as he prepares to play the real-life part of the cheated husband with his young wife. My mom took my hand in hers and squeezed it as she reached out and pressed a kiss in my hair. I had one arm around her frail shoulder and felt her whole body starting to shiver, so I covered her knees with her favorite blue blanket. At those heartrending words "Laugh, Pulcinello," and the sob of anguish from the very depths of his being, our tears flowed as freely as his.

I hadn't felt so close to my mother in years; we were once again united by our shared memories.

31

Changing Fashions

AT THE END OF 1998, Germaine's health had improved somewhat, and since she'd been cooped up for months, we were all eager
to have an outing together before the worst of winter closed in.
When Germaine received an invitation to a fashion show—just the
kind of event that was sure to appeal to her—we seized the opportunity.

The designer, Fong Leng, always put on exotic and colorful
shows, and the jet set of Amsterdam would put in an appearance
during what promised to be a fun afternoon. Germaine was looking forward to the treat, and the weather, though wet, was mild.
Hetty, who had known Fong Leng for years, was delighted to join
us. She also hadn't been out on the town in quite a while: she put
on her brightest clothes for the occasion and dusted off her video
camera.

We wrapped Germaine in a warm coat, stowed her wheelchair
in my car, and off we went. I was so proud: perfectly made up, and
with her hair neatly styled, she still retained something of her old

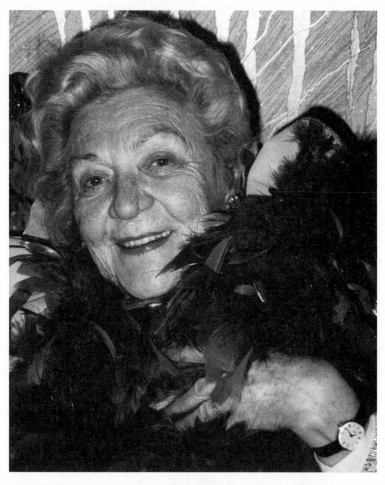

Still stylish

elegance. With us was an old friend, a handsome Indonesian
caterer who had long adored my mother. Ever the gentleman, he
arrived with two splendid bouquets, one for Fong Leng and the
other for Germaine. The show was held in the Frisia Museum, a
monumental building half an hour's drive outside the city. As her
wheelchair passed through the crowded lobby, quite a few old

friends greeted my mom, among them some of Mick's former patients. At one point she was reunited with a very special friend, her hairdresser of twenty-five years ago; there were tears in the old man's eyes as he grasped her hand.

The show was a great success: Germaine radiated happiness, her aches and pains forgotten until the time came for us to leave. Hetty and I would gladly have stayed longer, but when it became clear that Germaine was getting very tired, we made our way to the exit.

Our friend the caterer had parked the car at the corner of the street. He'd left his coat hanging in the cloakroom, with the keys in it; now he asked us to wait while he fetched it and said good-bye to some friends.

Outside, though, it was raining hard; we had no umbrella, and it had turned freezing cold. I urged him to hurry. Germaine was pale and shivering by the time we got her to the car.

Less than a week later Hetty phoned me.

"Come at once," she said, sobbing. "Your mother has been rushed to the hospital. She has double pneumonia. The doctor wants to talk to you urgently."

I HAD HAD an uncomfortable encounter at my mom's home just two days after that ill-fated show. My mother, I thought, had always accepted my unorthodox life with aplomb; she had weathered the shock of my former career and accepted the partners with whom I had developed stable relationships, from my husband, Paul, and later John, even down to Romke and Dia, whom she warmed up to over time. So I never expected that the news of a new lover in my life would upset her. Now, unthinkingly, I chattered on to her blithely all about Pauline, a bright and creative artist and musician and a perfect sexual match for me. But Germaine cut me off abruptly.

"What about Dia?"

I explained that we were going through a rough patch right now and launched back into my celebration of Pauline: she was ten years younger than Dia; we had so much fun together; she made me laugh.

Germaine was outraged. "I've had it with your endless parade of exciting new lovers, male or female," she snapped. She was seriously distressed: I noticed beads of sweat on her brow, and her breath was ragged. "I am an old woman. I certainly do not want to hear any more details of your intimate life. The only thing I want in my life now is to see you settle down and be happy with just one person who really cares for you. Yesterday it was Dia; today this Pauline. Who tomorrow? Stop behaving like a butterfly.

"I have grown fond of Dia. She is a good girl, and a serious person who loves you. So why can't you be sensible and stick to her? Now I think you should leave, and come back after you've broken with this Pauline and made up with Dia."

At that moment Hetty came in with a pot of tea, but Germaine ordered her to show me the door. For the umpteenth time, I was thrown out of my mother's house.

I WAS IN THAT STATE of disgrace when I got that distress call from Hetty. A reporter was interviewing me at the time, and she knew at once that something was wrong. I had just told her that I had been so traumatized as a child in the war that I was unable to cry, and now my tears were uncontrollable. I explained that I had to leave immediately for the hospital, but she kept pressing me for more time, firing questions at me about my mother.

"Please, I must ask you to go now," I pleaded. "Can't you see this is an emergency? My mom is old and weak, and she might well die." With these words I pushed her out of the door; she had barely a chance to grab her bags and cassette recorder.

"Can't I stay here and get the news firsthand—you know, about her death?" she asked.

I slammed the door and ran upstairs to remove my smearing makeup and put on some comfortable clothes. Then I rushed out the door to be with my mother.

32

Swan Song

(Germaine's Narrative)

It took Hetty and Xaviera quite a bit of convincing to persuade me to go to the Fong Leng show. It had been so long since I had
left the house. Fong Leng is something of a household name in the
Dutch fashion world. She was flamboyant and eloquent, an elegant
Chinese woman of indefinite age, immaculately made up and dressed
in her own exquisite, very expensive outfits, always designed with color
and flair. Hetty had been her friend for twenty-five years, and sometimes we squabbled over her exuberant enthusiasm for this powerful
woman, who had supposedly devoured dozens of attractive, young
female lovers. Her personality so dominated Hetty that she would
show up at every fashion show with her video camera to record the
event—not only for her own pleasure, but also to please Fong Leng,
to whom she would personally hand deliver a copy of the video soon
thereafter.

The show was held in the Frisia Museum, a relatively new museum
about twenty minutes from my house. It was an astonishing spectacle.

Multicolored patchwork coats, vividly presented on mannequins and live models alike. The alabaster skin of the exquisite models, among them a number of Indonesian girls, contrasted dramatically with the bright colors of the display as they paraded up and down the ramp with an allure and feline grace I had not seen for years. It brought me back to my own days modeling in Amsterdam, when people would applaud as I passed in one of Max Heymans's latest extravaganzas.

Hetty, Fong Leng's lifelong fan, was in her element. With Xaviera there to look after me, I had resolved not to be possessive and gave Hetty freedom to flit around, taking pictures and filming to her heart's content. Of course I kept an eye on her, and every fifteen minutes or so she would come back to where I was sitting and bring me a cup of coffee or a piece of cake. Wim, my hairdresser from years gone by, managed to slip me two glasses of my favorite medium dry sherry while Hetty's back was turned.

Hetty made a charming short and emotional speech, while she and her friend offered the diva an enormous bouquet of flowers. Standing beside me, looking radiant in one of Fong Leng's outfits, my child gently squeezed my hand and winked at Hetty when she had finished her speech. Xaviera and her caterer friend maneuvered me through the crowds all afternoon, but eventually my head started spinning, and I couldn't take it any longer.

I was very tired suddenly, and wanted nothing more than to be home in my own bed with a nice cup of coffee. But I didn't want to spoil their fun, so I gave Xaviera and her caterer friend an extra half an hour, though I was feeling weaker by the minute and beginning to shiver. I had sat next to an open door and it had been quite drafty. As I waited, I thought back to those days at my hairdresser's. How he would fuss over my long hair, pinning it up in a Grace Kelly chignon; what care he would take to keep the shade of blond Mick liked so much. The stories we told each other, the confessions we made: they were enough to fill a book.

I remember telling him how Mick loved to take me to the Moulin Rouge, where we would watch those gorgeous girls kicking their legs

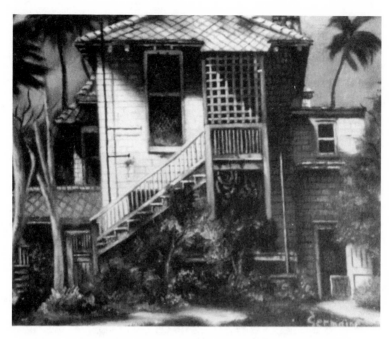

Germaine's painting of an Indonesian house

into the air and showing off their frilly knickers. Back in Amsterdam I would practice in front of our full-length bedroom mirror while Mick was paying his house calls. When he came home and was ready for bed, I would surprise my man with his own cancan show, for him alone. A command performance for one! And how excited he would get. I could kick as high as any of them—and who needs frilly panties anyway?

Ah, my legs in my younger years: my pride and glory. Unlike Dietrich, I never bothered to have them insured for a million dollars, but they were seductively long, and agile, and I was so proud of them, sheathed in the sheerest silk.

How weak and wasted I felt as I sat, helpless, in that wheelchair, waiting in the freezing drizzle for the car. At least I have left Xaviera the memory of her mother, dancing passionately for her father.

AND NOW, barely a week later, I find myself in the hospital. I had waited too long for the farewells.

I must have dozed off, weakened as I am by painkillers, for I just saw Mick's face in front of me, just as he used to look before his body was ravaged by illness. We were back at LiLaLo, a Yiddish cabaret; he was swapping yarns with the couple who ran the place. And there was Julius and his wife, and Mick and I were playing gin rummy with them. But dreams turn to nightmares: Mick on his deathbed, in torment. Why couldn't they let him die in peace and with dignity, instead of tearing out his teeth, as if that could do any good? His cheeks sagged; his whole face seemed to collapse.

I awoke in a panic. Will some officious young doctor come by to pull out my last teeth, leave me to suffer the same agony? No—Xaviera won't let them do that to me. Teeth! I remember the trick I played on Hetty. She was eager to go to a carnival in her native town, but I didn't want to go and didn't want her going on her own. I suppose I must have resented the idea that she was prepared to leave me behind to go and enjoy herself. So I put her false teeth in a plastic bag and hid them in a garbage bin. I can still remember her, all dressed up and ready to go, growing more and more puzzled as she looked for her dentures. I knew she was far too vain to go without them. Of course, I eventually confessed—after it was too late. She really didn't react too badly, once she got over her disappointment. She knew that if I didn't allow her to go, it was because I loved her so much that I couldn't let her out of my sight. At least I think that's how she saw it. She seldom wears her dentures around the house these days—they hurt her gums—though most of the time when Xaviera comes she quickly inserts them. I'm used to her silly face without those teeth, though I certainly don't want to look like that. Still, I sometimes wonder how I will look when I die.

I worry more about what I will die of. I remember one macabre conversation I had with Xaviera not that long ago. She had been worrying about the same thing, frightened that my end would be painful and humiliating. She reminded me of the screams of the old woman who lived upstairs when Mick first started his practice in Amsterdam. She had been ill for years—and then to hear that final scream, the agony of her death! That was years ago, but I can still hear it in my head. I dread being struck by a series of strokes like Mick. Maybe a heart attack, then a few hours of pain? I suggested that to Xaviera, but she said I was far too tough for my heart to give out. I suppose she was being kind, hoping to reassure me. But what if it is something worse? I often wake up choking, gasping for breath, and I fear I will die that way.

So they have given me an inhaler—a puffer, I call it—and they are letting me go home. Well, at least it won't be pneumonia that kills me off. I'll be glad to be out of this gloomy hospital, but what have I got to look forward to? Unable to move a step on my own, Hetty bossing me about, not even letting me have a little drink. As much as I hated losing my breasts, losing my independence was worse. I am glad my child has been around so much lately; in fact I doubt if she ever left the city this last year. Poor girl: she loves traveling so much and gave all that up to be with her mother. But even speaking with her is an effort now.

WHY CAN'T I be left to die in peace! How long ago was it that I was sent home from that awful hospital? I can't remember; time seems to get jumbled in my tired old brain. But what am I doing in the hospital again?

It was Hetty's fault. She had filled my hot water bottle and was squeezing out the air when the phone rang. I insisted that the water always be scalding hot. Xaviera used to make a fuss about it, but I was the one with the pains in my stomach. Trying to help me take a little walk around the room while she was grabbing the phone at the same time, Hetty lost hold of me, and that's how I came to fall smack onto the open hot water bottle as I sat back on the couch. We had both forgotten that the top hadn't been screwed on, and I was scorched. I didn't have much meat left to burn anyway; I'd become extremely skinny, almost ghostlike. It was a second-degree burn, and it was agony. It left an enormous blister that had to be looked after carefully for weeks.

When the accident happened, Xaviera was on the other end of the phone, and all she could hear were my screams of pain. My child was worried silly. Hetty had of course instantly turned her attention to me and forgotten about the dangling phone with her on the other end. Luckily Xaviera showed up soon after, and so did the doctor.

But no, that was all weeks ago. It must have been something else. It must have been the pains in my stomach and my back that made them bring me here.

They give me strong painkillers. My only relief comes when I drift into sleep. They make me quite woozy, and when I open my eyes, I am not sure at first where I am. Xaviera is sitting beside the bed with someone next to her. It's not Hetty … yes, I recognize Dia. I smile at them, but I am too weak to talk. Hardly surprising, since for two days the doctors had emptied my stomach and then stuck that endoscope right up into it. I had dreaded that, but the pain and discomfort were less extreme than when I had undergone the same examination years ago. Old age dulls the senses.

There was no need for this ordeal. How many times had I made Hetty take me to a hospital since they chopped off my breasts? I knew the cancer had come back: the learned doctors told me I was wrong. Now their verdict, after the examination and all the X rays, was that my stomach lining is full of polyps. They avoided using the word *cancer*, but I knew. I had always known.

"You must eat to keep up your strength." I gaze at the nurse. I am dying, and they want me to keep my strength up! The food is horrible; my appetite has disappeared. I chewed smaller and smaller pieces, but it was difficult. So when I had the strength, I would spit out the half-chewed, nauseating morsels and hide them. Once Xaviera walked in and caught me: she was furious and told me off, as though I were a ten-year-old kid found cheating.

I CLOSE MY EYES and hear Xaviera walk into the corridor. She is talking with the young doctor who examined me. I may be too weak to speak, but don't they realize I can still hear?

"We can do nothing more, madam. Her condition is too far gone. And your mother is too weak to survive another operation. I think it best if we let her have a room of her own for her last few days." I have been in a room with six other patients.

NOW THAT THE DOCTORS have given up hope for me, they have ceased mauling my frail body, and I am enjoying longer periods of consciousness. Strange how memory works. Xaviera came and read me some of my favorite poems: Goethe, Schiller, Heine—things I had learned as a schoolgirl, and I remembered them perfectly. I believe I even recited a few out loud with her: soothing words in German, my mother tongue, which I had almost forgotten. Yet things that happened last week are lost in a fog of oblivion.

Even more bizarre, they have wheeled in a new patient, an Indonesian, and placed him in a bed next to mine. He was obviously scared, so I made a great effort to speak a few words to him. Without any conscious effort I addressed him in Malay, a language I hadn't used for almost forty years. But later that afternoon Dia was talking to me, and it was all too much effort. My mind blanked out. I've heard people speak of long-term memory gain and short-term memory loss in old age. What was my age anyway? For so long I have told little white lies about it that now I have really forgotten what year I was born. I do remember it was the second of May, and that Mick's birthday was the eighteenth of February.

I could not follow the conversation. I couldn't remember the last words Dia said. She and Xaviera had stopped talking. They could see from my expression that I was no longer with them.

XAVIERA SAYS that my nephew Harold is coming to see me. Of course from Mick's side of the family only Carry, a niece, showed up with her husband. Her mother was dead, and her father had not been on speaking terms with me for many years. Carry had always been fond of me and especially of Mick. But when her parents had read about Xaviera's call-girl agency in the papers, they had been quite upset. The only one I got on with was Arthur, and he was long dead. Beppy, Arthur's wife, who liked to appear so broad-minded, had bought a copy of *The Happy Hooker;* after she read it, she burned it and sent me the ashes in the post with a letter telling me she wanted no further contact with my daughter or with me either.

Suddenly I was a pariah. Didn't they have any sympathy for how I would suffer? Didn't they think of the scorn, the taunts of self-righteous neighbors? The only one who stood by me was dear old Julius, and he wasn't even a blood relation.

I was so ashamed—not by the book, but by my daughter having been guilty of such disgraceful behavior. Thank God her father never knew the full truth of the years she spent in New York. I told her that once, and she replied that if he had been alive, none of it might have happened. She would have had no reason to flee the country, to escape the grief of confronting her dying father.

But I was not going to turn my back on her now, when she was being attacked on all sides. And, in truth, I had a grudging admiration for the businesslike way she had handled her affairs. And when I read the book myself, I had to admit it was honest, and I have always admired honesty. I had been so strict with her when she was a child. Perhaps I should take some credit.

Credit? Am I not the one who should take the blame? She had gone to a good school, and I had forced my ideas of morality on her. So if she had gone off the rails, it must have been my fault. Where had I gone wrong? I should have been ashamed not of Xaviera but of myself. I had failed her as a mother. Now I agonize over every dispute, every quarrel, but I don't know what I should have done differently. Had I been too strict, forced her into revolt? I don't know, and anyway it is too late.

I am not ashamed of my daughter. No, I am proud of her.

THEY SAY THAT on one's deathbed one's past life flashes before one. When I was desperately ill with pneumonia, I kept seeing before my eyes my beloved Mick, in health and in sickness. But now, as my time runs out, it is not the past but the future that haunts me. When I am no longer there, who will watch over Xaviera? She has fallen for some smooth talkers in her time. I suspected everybody. If only she had settled down with some man with a sound head on his shoulders. Now she seems happy with Dia, and she has a sweet nature. But will she be tough-minded enough to save Xaviera from her own impulsiveness? And who next will she take into her bed, or bring into her life? I am glad I lived long enough to see her make a success of something else in her life, to see her prove wrong all those petty prudes who said she lived only for sex. It does me good to see how well respected her theater has become.

I worry over her health. She tends to eat too fast and too much. Maybe that is my fault as well. What should I have done to help her live the life of a contented and fulfilled woman?

Sleep: I am too tired. Worry exhausts me. If only Mick were here. How upset he was when I tricked him into making me pregnant! But how he loved Xaviera when she was born! I knew he wanted a son, and I remember my anguish at the fact that I was giving him a girl. He had already chosen Xavier as the name of our firstborn.

Of course, that's it. Now I see where I went wrong. Why did I never give Xaviera a brother? There was plenty of time—but I was mean to Mick. His silly little affairs made me bitter, so not giving him a son was my way of punishing him. And the one who suffered was Xaviera. Her childhood might have been so different; her love for her father might never have been so obsessive, her jealousy of me so strong. And by now there would have been a man in her life to help and guide her. With all her friends and lovers, I can feel her loneliness. She will miss me.

ONE MORE DAY. Harold has been and gone. Hetty has just dozed off in her chair at the end of my bed. She has wept so much. I am sure she will miss me a lot when I am no longer here. Now I feel remorse because I did not tell her often enough how much I cared for her, something she always craved to hear from my lips. I don't know what held me back; I am not as extroverted as Xaviera, and words just don't come easy.

The room is growing so dark, but I can feel Xaviera at my side. I think Dia is with her, but I do not see clearly anymore. I sense the presence of my child; I can smell her own fragrance, and now she has just put a handkerchief drenched in some 4711 eau de cologne between my fingers. That smell brings back a flash of my mother's sweet face on her own deathbed, the woman who could not cry, and whom I have missed as much as Vera will miss me. My child, my flesh and blood. There is no one in the world I have loved more, much as it may have upset Hetty. No one could ever come between my daughter and me, even when we fought—how I suffered the times I sent her away, how often I wished I had bitten my tongue.

Xaviera has placed her hand ever so gently on mine. It is almost too much, but I no longer have strength even to move my hands or any other part of my body. It is as though my body is no longer mine. I no longer feel any guilt or regret. My daughter has brought me peace. She has been here with me until the very end, as she promised.

I can still hear all that goes on around me. Xaviera must have called Hetty, and there are two nurses beside my bed. My breathing picks up; the setting sun is shining on my face; I feel warm and mellow; but suddenly I cannot stop my chest heaving. My heart is pumping the blood into my brain faster and faster. Colors start appearing, beautiful colors, red and orange like blood, and purple and white like the clouds I saw just before I started this final journey. I seem to have opened my eyes, or so

Xaviera says, but I am not aware of my actions anymore. Apparently I am staring at the ceiling, and she is surprised to see my eyes so wide and open and beautiful. The word *heavenly* escapes from her mouth in a whisper. I hear the muffled cries of my child, and in the distance I can hear Hetty too. Then there is the calm voice of the young nurse, whom I can no longer see, but whose voice I recognize. She feels my pulse....

"It's about time for your mother to leave us—just a few more moments," she says.

Her older colleague adds: "So harmonious, you three around her. So much love between you all. Something we seldom see."

Then my child's voice near my ear: "Mammi, please take it easy. Slow down, let go. You may go now. We all love you. We are all with you."

Her tears fall onto my cheeks, but I cannot kiss her anymore. I am too far gone already.

Total peace and happiness envelop me. I feel free at last, free of pain and sorrow, though I can no longer look after my *piekeltje*. A child no more.

33

The Long Farewell

DIA SPENT the next few nights with me, comforting me in her protective and reassuring arms. But both of us were tearful. It was as though part of her had died, she told me; she had been orphaned for ten years; then, desperately missing her own mother, she had found herself a new family in mine. That night she suggested a title for the book I was writing: *Kind Af,* which translates as *Child No More.* "We are the next generation on death row," she said, falling into one of her black moods. I nodded and cried some more.

I had begun writing again not long before, while my mother was spending her very last few days in the hospital and I was sitting beside her. While she slept I worked on a piece that would become her eulogy; when I finished, I read her the words slowly and clearly, with tears staining my face. She was able to understand it all, and when I reached the end, she took my hand in hers and pressed a kiss on it. "Veraatje, *kindje*," she said softly, "you must really love me more than I had ever thought, to devote so many words to your dying mother and write such loving things about me and your father." She reached up for me to kiss her face. She was warm and feverish; the strain of listening had tired her.

She paused; I gave her some water. There was something more she wanted to say before going to sleep. Her words came out ever so softly now, and I had to put my ear to her mouth to understand her.

"You know, my *piekeltje*, I always knew you could write well, and not only about sex. How long has it been since you published your last book?"

"About twelve years," I answered. "Ever since John told me I couldn't write my way out of a paper bag, I've been suffering some kind of writer's block."

"Nonsense—he is full of rubbish." She seemed to regain some strength and laughed wryly. "You can write, and I have the feeling there is a lot more you want to write about once I am gone. Go ahead, you have my blessing, as long as you don't hurt anybody with it. I hope it will be totally different from anything you have so far written."

And that is how the spell was lifted and I began to write this book.

THE MORNING after she passed I woke at five. My biological clock had switched: I used to go to sleep around four and wake up at eight, but in the hospital I had been falling asleep around midnight and waking at the crack of dawn. I sensed something in the room move ever so lightly, rustling the curtains, and suddenly felt that the spirit of my mother had entered my bedroom. It was as if she had opened the curtains just a bit, to peep around the corner and wish me good morning.

Then, three days later, Dia and a few other close friends had dinner in my garden, as the weather was splendid. Dia was setting the table when there was a sudden gust of wind. All the trees and plants swayed violently; then the wind stopped as suddenly as it had started, and again I sensed my mother's presence. She always liked trees; she'd told me they had a life of their own, and believed they were possessed by spirits. Now I could almost hear her: "Have a nice meal. I'll be watching over you all. Enjoy!"

Another dear friend, the very talented American artist Mark van Holden, came by. We seldom met, but whenever we did, there was a great meeting of the minds and the warmth of friendship. Mark is a rare human being, noble, considerate, and spiritual, and some-how he always shows up when I need him most, without my call-ing. That night he handed me *The Tibetan Book of Living and Dying* by Sogyal Rinpoche. Inside he had put a picture: a scene of sky, pink and orange, shading to purple, with soft white clouds—exactly what I had dreamed when I thought I was dying myself, and probably the very scene reflected in my mother's eyes.

EVERY WEEK I used to go swimming close to Zorgvlied. Next Tuesday, I would return: Zorgvlied is the huge cemetery where my mom long ago reserved a plot, deep inside the expanse of green lawns. But as death approached she instructed Hetty to pay an extra thousand guilders to move her plot to a space close to the entrance, to make her resting place more accessible for me.

I discovered this only when I met the undertaker, who treated me with great kindness as we completed the paperwork. I was asked to choose everything: a color and lining for the coffin, the details of catering and flowers, the timing and recording of speeches in the hall, right down to whether I wanted the coffin carried to the grave manually or mechanically.

It was all too great a strain; I tried to control my tears, so as not to be embarrassed. But the undertaker, a warmhearted man, noticed my distress and urged me not to hold back just to spare their feelings. There was no need to hurry, so I gave way to a fit of sobbing before coming back to the business details. The only thing that had been paid for was the burial plot, but I assured him that I would spare no reasonable expense so that everything would proceed easily. In two hours, everything she had desired had been done: a white coffin, covered with red roses and green foliage by Hetty and our many mutual friends, enhanced by an enormous bunch of white lilies, interspersed with red roses, and our picture.

After giving the undertaker the text for the obituary notices, I asked a final favor: that I be allowed to help with my mother's makeup before the viewing.

He made a few phone calls, gave us the addresses we would need, and warned me not to be put off by the appearance of the bearded old man who was the makeup artist.

Later, after tending to other arrangements, we went to the new funeral parlor, situated in an idyllic woodland setting. The bearded man was waiting for us and brought us tea. In the bright sunshine my mother looked perfectly at peace, and he remarked on her beauty, saying he could not believe that this was a woman in her mid-eighties. Her skin was so smooth that he suggested I might not need to apply makeup to so exquisite a face.

But I knew my mom well enough to know she would appreciate a touch of glamour, even in her very last moments on earth. So I had brought with me some gray-blue eye shadow, her favorite brown eyebrow pencil, a little lip liner, a soft pinkish orange lipstick, dark blue mascara, and some rouge.

In passing, the makeup artist told me he was actually an artist— a still-life painter, of all things. I asked why he didn't prefer working on living people rather than the dead.

"But what I do is such relaxed and gratifying work. You see, as a painter I am good with quiet things. If only you knew how many bodies are brought here in a dreadful state: it is wonderful to be complimented by their families when they see their beloved looking again as they did in life." He was a sweet man with a gentle nature.

As we worked together, I felt my mother's icy skin, kissed the side of her nose, and touched her forehead, then lifted her neatly folded fingers a fraction and pulled the scarf out from underneath her hands, wrapping it the way she would have. When I looked at her once more, I felt I could almost see her chest move up and down, as though she were still breathing.

All that was left to do was spray some Chanel No. 5 into her coffin, and help put on a pair of favorite earrings I had given her: she always felt naked without them.

Still there were two more days to go: tonight the body on display, the ceremony itself at midday tomorrow.

THE FUNERAL WAS an elaborate but tasteful affair, just as Germaine would have wanted. The weather was fine, and at least seventy-five people must have been in attendance. The tension was palpable, voices low and hushed, many tears shed. Half the people who attended were younger friends of mine; the rest were older, friends and acquaintances of Hetty and Germaine, most of them from Oss, where they had spent a great deal of time. Seldom have I seen so many youngish people paying homage to a woman of such advanced age.

The music I chose carefully: from the spiritual tranquillity of a Mahler *adagietto* to the simple sentiment of songs touchingly rendered by Karin Bloemen and Cleo Laine. Those who knew her best and would miss her most expressed their tributes in farewell speeches. My own words dwelt on so many events in the lives of my parents and myself, and on the personalities that made up the story of our lives together. Dia and Romke spoke movingly of their fond memories. Finally, Carry added her valedictory; apart from myself, she was the only member of our family to speak. She reminded us of the sarcasm and insults Germaine had suffered from some of Mick's family because of her German parentage, but also reminded us that her loyalty and devotion to her husband had never wavered.

In her elegant black dress and high heels, Carry had a sophisticated charm that contrasted vividly with Hetty's earthy style. Yet it was Hetty's simple directness that made perhaps the greatest impression, and not only on me. Knowing that she wasn't accustomed to making formal speeches, I had advised her to make some notes the day before the ceremony, and she walked to the podium with a paper in her hand, with which she fumbled as she started hesitantly to speak. But soon her emotions gave her eloquence as she unfolded for us her story of the happiness and the sadness of her life with Germaine. She thanked me for the pains I had taken to ensure this occasion would be worthy of my mom, and then we shared her anguish as she told of the emptiness in her heart. At the end she turned and showed us the paper she was holding: it was completely blank. "I speak from my heart," she said, "that needs no written text."

Before the coffin was closed we had a last chance to look at Germaine. Her face now spoke of death; the makeup had worn off. Gently, Hetty dropped rose petals over her eyes, but there was something uncomfortable about witnessing her now. Perhaps she had remained unburied a day too long. I shall try to remember her face as it was the day before.

DIA HAD BEEN with me for almost a week: now she went home to resume her own life. She had provided wonderful support to Hetty and me during these most difficult days of our lives, but now she needed a break.

Dia had newly acquired cats to look after, and so did I. When I came back from the funeral, I felt empty and lonely, no matter how many dear friends tried to comfort me. About six months before, though, I had brought two tiny kittens from Spain—one black, the other gray. I am particularly fond of Spanish cats; when neutered, they tend to remain smaller than Dutch cats, which can grow large and lethargic. The two kittens were cute but rather wild and untamable. I particularly fancied the gray one but had given neither one a name: the black one was usually called Blackie, but the gray one remained an enigma, running shyly away when anyone tried to approach him.

On that sad day, though, I went upstairs to take a much-needed nap in the late afternoon. And there, sitting on my bed, was this beautiful gray kitten, looking at me with his head tilted as if to plead with me: "Please stroke me. Rub my neck. I am all yours at last." For once he didn't run away but began to purr the moment my hand touched his soft fur, and seemed to ask for more. His affectionate purr recalled my mom looking at me so lovingly that last time I stroked her neck and shoulders. How I enjoyed rubbing ever so gently the back of my hand against her neck and hair. It was as though I could still feel her quiver with happiness, joy radiating from my fingers as they rubbed her neck and massaged her tired head. When I went to remove my hand, she purred much like the cat and wordlessly begged me to continue. With my eyes closed, for a few moments it was as if my own mother had come back to life.

THE DAY after her funeral, I went over to my mom's place and started taking to pieces the flat where she had been living for the last thirty years. Putting books into boxes, sorting out photographs and knickknacks, most of all touching her dresses and the little hats she used to wear: it all filled me with sadness. There were lovely handbags, little boxes and wallets with notes and pictures, letters from me years and years old, all sorts of mementos. I put her lipstick and cosmetics and her jewelry into boxes, and had difficulty stopping my tears as I recalled occasions when she wore them. For myself I assembled a box full of her soft silk and crepe de chine scarves, some of which still held her fragrance. Of course I will treasure them, will go on wearing them and breathing their perfume.

ONCE THE FIRST SHOCK of loss had begun to wear off, I gained some control over my tears. Where once I cried three times a day, soon I cried once every three days. The smallest things

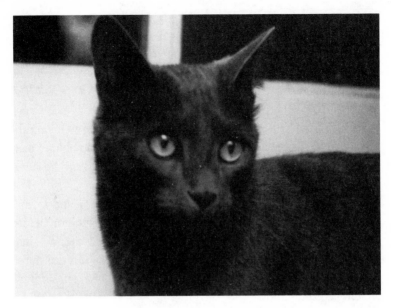

The gray kitten

reminded me of her: a visit to a café where we used to spend our afternoons, a shopkeeper asking after her, unaware of her death.

Then came a more bizarre evocation of her spirit. The gray kitten went missing, and for a moment it was almost a second bereavement. But then Dia and I were sitting around the table in my living room one night when a strange apparition crept slowly through the cat flap. Almost twice the size of my cats, coated in a thick mass of gray mud, it seemed a veritable symbol of death.

Then, beneath this filth, I recognized my gray kitten. He walked up to me and stood motionless before my feet; his once-glossy fur was covered in what looked to be so dense a layer of clay that he could hardly move a paw. There was a cement mixer down the road; he must have fallen in, and the cement was rapidly hardening around his body. I panicked: he seemed to be mummifying before my eyes. But Dia immediately sprang into action. We filled the bathtub, and Dia shampooed the struggling cat as thoroughly as she could while I held him still. Eventually we got him clean enough to bring him to the vet, but his eyes were still closed and full of grit, and it took her a good two hours to finish the job. Though now he has finally recovered, for the next two weeks he could barely manage to open his eyes.

AMONG THE BYSTANDERS on the path that led to my mother's idyllic resting place had been one strange face, an elderly man with glasses. His expression was kind and thoughtful, and he stood a discreet distance from the crowd of mourners.

A few days later, while visiting her grave again, Dia and I came across the man once more, standing as if in silent meditation before an extraordinary grave. A multicolored glass sculpture stood amid lovely flowers and candlesticks, and in front of it was a metal statue of a naked woman, her belly and breasts arched high, as if to encompass the sculpted globe.

We learned that Cor, as he was called, had created this beautiful work of art to commemorate his beloved wife, who had died the year before, and not a day passed without his visiting this shrine. Whenever I made my midday pilgrimage to my mother's grave I was sure to meet him, and he became a close friend. He would talk to his wife as if she were still alive; he wrote poetry for her, and took a beautiful series of pictures of the cemetery in summer and winter. It was hard to believe that they had been taken at Zorgvlied, these dreamlike photos of a rabbit or a pheasant sitting on a tombstone; they seemed almost to have been taken in a tropical rain forest or a jungle. His dead wife had become his muse.

Never having been inspired by the conventions of cemetery monuments, I asked him to design a grave sculpture for my mother. What I wanted would be smaller and simpler than what he had constructed for his wife, rendered in glowing warm colors, symbolic of the mutual love of mother and daughter. Cor was no businessman, and I knew he would welcome a few thousand guilders. After some consideration, he consented.

It would be finished and placed in the spring of the year 2000, the season of life renewed.

34

Sorrow Knows No Frontiers

SOME TIME after my mother's death, on a much-needed vacation in Zihuatenejo, Mexico, with Dia and John, I was awakened by the wails of a weeping woman. Our neighbor, a sixty-five-year-old Canadian woman, had learned that day that her favorite son had been found dead by friends. He had probably suffered a heart attack or a stroke, and his body, already beginning to decompose, had lain undiscovered for ten days. Her husband was flying to Edmonton to identify the body and authorize an autopsy. I had met the young man a few years earlier and found him a sweet person—perhaps too good for this world.

All the local residents had come to offer their condolences, but now the poor woman was left utterly alone. Her sobs kept Dia and me awake all night and cut through each fiber of my being. In the morning I saw her on her veranda, her eyes red and swollen: she had aged ten years overnight. I went to her and took her trembling body in my arms. She seemed to have shrunk, and I hugged her slender body tight. In a voice hoarse from weeping, she moaned, "You know what it is to lose someone dear to you, don't you, Xaviera? I saw how you cried when you told us that your mom had died. She was so dear to you." She had to pause to choke down her tears. "It's just not fair that a child should go before its parents. It is just not fair!"

I could no longer hold back my own tears. Then she cried out, "Please, Xaviera, tell me, how long does this mourning take? I just can't seem to stop crying."

I comforted her as best I could, and clasped her in my arms. "Give it as long as it takes and you'll slowly begin to work yourself out of the sorrow. And then the healing process will start, or so I hope. You see, I lost my mom only half a year ago."

The following morning my whole body felt heavy: I could barely open my eyes, and to climb out of bed was absolutely impossible. I knew I hadn't suffered a heart attack or a stroke, but agonizing pains racked my stomach, much as they had my mother's in her last few years of life.

When Dia woke up, she was surprised that I didn't leap out of bed as usual. She gave me a gentle push, but I didn't stir. Alarmed, she gazed at my glassy eyes and ran to alert John, who was still sound asleep.

They bent over and shook me, but there was no way I could raise my limbs.

"She looks ashen," Dia said. "Only yesterday she was developing a tan."

I could barely keep my eyes open; a severe pain suddenly stabbed at my heart.

"What did she eat yesterday?" John asked, ever the practical man. "Or drink? Maybe she had some polluted water."

"No," I whispered. "It's nothing like that." I spoke with difficulty, and I could see the panic in their eyes as they sensed their helplessness. I begged them to go and leave me alone for a couple of hours, as I wanted to sleep some more. But I did anything but sleep. All that morning I writhed in torment, as moments of my life flashed through my mind. And I seemed to relive every pain my

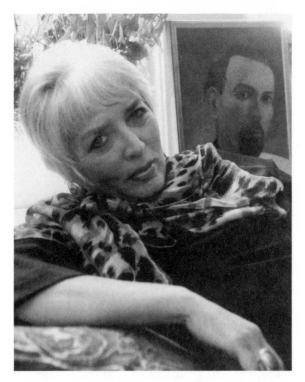

With a portrait of Mick

mother had ever suffered. It was as though I myself were dying, but inside her body.

Later, with difficulty, I managed to explain the feeling to Dia, who of course wanted to call for a doctor. I knew the only cure was time—if I should survive at all.

Eventually I convinced her, and she persuaded John to leave me to resolve this crisis alone. From time to time they looked in and brought me water, but it was two full days before it was over.

On the third morning, I awoke refreshed. It was as though I had come out of a protracted nightmare. But it had been no nightmare: rather, I had just found a way to know what my mother had gone through before the relief of death.

Epilogue

I TWICE VISITED the glass factory with Cor and selected the stained glass, orange, red, blue, and yellow, for the monument on my mother's grave. His design was of red and orange semicircles, symbols of mother and daughter rising from blue clouds: it was abstract but expressive, its message clear.

Hetty disapproved; she had always wanted a plain, black tombstone with the word GERMAINE engraved in gold letters. So she had a small, round stone manufactured, which I allowed to be placed in front of Cor's sculpture, far enough removed not to spoil the effect. That was Hetty's niche, with a little picture of my mother in a weatherproof metal frame, set between the branches of a diminutive metal bonsai tree and framed by plants she placed there in regular tribute.

For the unveiling of the memorial I invited a group of sixteen of my closest friends, all of whom had known Germaine. But there were two absentees. Hetty refused to come, for no particular reason, which hurt me quite a bit. And Romke stayed away too. He had paid his own homage to my mother, he said, "making her bed" by faithfully tending her garden at the cemetery. He was too private a person to endure yet another ceremony. Like Hetty, he had already said his farewell in his own way.

But Romke was there when the men came to mount the sculpture firmly in place, forever to mark my mother's final resting place. As soon as the earth had been replaced, he rearranged the surrounding greenery to showcase and complement its beauty.

It was slightly overcast during the ceremony, but at the moment of the unveiling the sun broke through the clouds, bathing the whole scene with radiant light. Behind stood two young rosebushes Romke had recently planted: in a year's time they will look magnificent.

For Dia and me, each trip to the graveyard was a delightful escape into tranquillity from the rat race of my life, as I worked to overcome my sorrow by producing yet more and more plays and drowning myself in work. Romke helped us by placing two red metal chairs from my garden right next to the grave, so whoever might come to visit could have a seat and relax, and we could open our hearts to my mother.

My mother once asked me, "Veraatje, when I die, please take a bench or a chair and go and sit down near me. Just ring the bell and wake me up so we can talk a bit." A good friend recently gave me a lovely Tibetan bell, which gives a wonderful sound when struck, and so now I shall place it nearby.

Spring is in the air. The view from your grave will be spectacular when the sun shines through Cor's sculpted glass vision. On his daily visit to his wife, he will no doubt walk past your grave and think of you. Dia and Romke will be there often. And I shall be there always, sitting by your side, so we can talk a bit.

Rest in peace.
Your loving flesh and blood, Veraatje
Child no more.

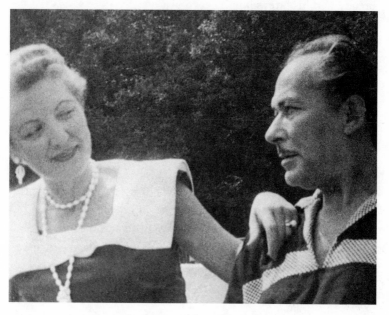

Germaine and Mick in love

Appendix:
Speech at the Graveside

GERMAINE: a beautiful French name for a woman who, even during her last moments on this earth, retained her French charm. That mixture of German *Tuechtigkeit* (strictness) and French flair was typical and always there.

All my mother's life she has had *das gewissene etwas* (that something very special about her) to deal with people, to make them feel at ease, like the way she stood for many years beside her husband, my father, Dr. Mick de Vries, in his practice as a doctor.

For her, there were no differences between class or background. But she was indeed critical of some people, especially those who used to come to the house, introduced by me—her daughter. She wanted nothing but the very best for me, the only child to whom she lovingly gave birth. I was conceived in love at a time when World War II was raging throughout Europe and threatening to break out in Indonesia, as well.

Shortly after my birth, we were all interned in concentration camps for the next three long years. There my parents were tortured, beaten, insulted, and treated more like lice than human beings.

My mother fought like a lioness to keep me alive. My father underwent severe torture, helping many sick women in an overcrowded women's camp. Trying to smuggle medications into the camp, he was tortured as punishment for his frequent heroic efforts to save the lives of his patients.

After the war, we were reunited and repatriated to Amsterdam. There Mick had to start from scratch at an age when most doctors would think of retiring. He, once a famous psychiatrist and director of a respected hospital in Surabaya, was now back to being a general practitioner again. Yet, in no time, people knew where to find him, and they came from all over Europe to see him and to be treated by him. He had that magic touch and was an excellent diagnostician, a doctor by vocation, not just in it for the money.

I have enjoyed much love bestowed on me in my youth and later on in life by both my parents. I have seen what it means for two people to love each other. It has taught me how to show love and affection to others. They educated me in an open and honest way, taught me the difference between right and wrong. I inherited a sense of humor from my father, as well as the aesthetic sense and intuition of my mother.

Even though I was the only child, our house was often the meeting place of many artistic and colorful friends and acquaintances of my parents.

Humor ist wenn mann trotzdem lacht were words Germaine lived by, words that gave her strength in all her adversities.

Where my father was an egocentric, eccentric, extrovert humorous man, an entertainer par excellence and, at times, a flirt, my mother remained the charming, occasionally cool hostess, usually rather in the background but always dignified and helpful. Many a patient was able to confide in her, knowing their secrets would be safe.

Yet she had something naughty about her, something risqué, that mother of mine. She was not only extremely beautiful, a top model in her youth, but later, as a mature woman, she was also a great dancer. Sometimes even in private she danced for me, her greatest admirer. I shall never forget her long "Blue Bell Girl" legs.

My mother had the most elegant hands and fingers I had ever seen on a woman, and I think once my mother had read my book *The*

Happy Hooker, she finally learned to understand my father's sometimes unusual desires—it was all part of foreplay and piquancy. In a
way she was glad someone finally had written such a book, and it
opened her eyes, even though it was after her husband had died. And
that is how mother and daughter grew up, almost like two close sisters.
We had not a single secret from each other and were able to trust each
other explicitly: we shared good as well as bad tidings in love and in
sorrow.

Our small family traveled quite a bit throughout Europe. My father
taught me a different language every weekend. My mother was an
extremely intuitive woman and a great storyteller. She was also a very
generous person with a big heart. She certainly had more patience with
people than either my father or me.

Of course, it hit us like a bolt from the blue when my father suddenly suffered a massive stroke at the age of sixty-one, which left him
paralyzed on one side. In the course of eight years, he changed from a
healthy, brilliant, charming raconteur to a tiny, wilted wreck, a mere
vegetable. I used to say: "He has gone from Dostoevsky to Lucille
Ball." No wonder I shed quite a few tears when many years later I
heard that Lucille Ball had died. It was as if part of my youth had died
with her. He suffered at least seven strokes over the years before he
finally closed his eyes for good.

But he had been ill for barely a year when I selfishly spread my
wings, leaving my mom to cope with this tragedy alone. I fled to South
Africa, where I moved in with my father's first child from his previous
marriage. A few years later, I moved to New York and wrote a much
read book, full of my notorious adventures. So not only did Germaine
have to look after an invalid husband for so many years on her own,
but she also had to deal with this enormous blow to her ego from all
the scandal-mongering press about her sinful daughter who had now
openly become the notorious Madame X.

Germaine often must have wondered, "Why me?" Why did she
deserve this double ordeal? Did she forgive me for the embarrassing
moments that people and press put her through when they asked
about her daughter? Yes, of course she did and HOW! She had to

fight once more for me, not to keep me alive like in the concentration camp, but to keep the image of me alive, that deep down I was still a good person. The few friends she still had, like my father's own sister and her husband in The Hague, considered this the last straw and refused to have anything more to do with her. After the death of my father, she passed six very lonely years. I was still away in Canada most of that time and she was virtually without any friends. The loneliness was almost too much for the woman who, for eight long years, pushed her husband around in a wheelchair and looked after him. Finally, there came some ray of sunshine into her life again when I introduced her to Hetty during my own birthday party.

Hetty was like a gift from heaven, loving, cheerful, optimistic, active, a woman with many hobbies and handy around the house but, most of all, caring and devoted—feelings Germaine had been deprived of for so long. The rest of the story most of you know by now. Whereas my father used to be a somewhat dominant, even overpowering, personality, Hetty was cooperative and helpful. Although sometimes a bit of a know-it-all, she was above all kindhearted and dead honest. She adored the ground my mother walked on, and that was great for Germaine's ego. Even when Germaine became somewhat unruly and difficult toward the end of her life, Hetty would always keep her on the pedestal she had created for her. My mother appeared to be someone rather distant, reserved and critical, but she had a lot of style. Hetty, more unsophisticated and sometimes boyish, was impulsive, spontaneous, and sympathetic. Together they made rather an odd couple.

Each year I would spend the month of May with them. It was Germaine's birthday on the second. The three of us would move to Marbella, and I would spend as much time with them as I could.

Hetty came from the south of Holland, where they celebrate carnival extensively each year, and she liked to party, play the clown, and cheer my mom up whenever she could. Hetty could make a veritable happening out of a simple birthday party. When she dressed up as a clown, Germaine would softly say to me with a smile on her face, "There she goes again, 'Ridi, Pagliaccio'—Laugh then, clown." And how we have laughed and loved each other for most of these years!

Hetty accepted the strong symbiotic bond that existed between mother and daughter, though she too had her jealous moments when I got praised instead of her. She often told me: "Vera, if I did not love you so much, it would have been more difficult for me to put up with your mom, as she seems to have three major stories in her life, her undying love for you and your father and her horror stories of the war."

Well, Hetty as well as me will have to continue life without Germaine. She reached a ripe old age, but it is never the right age for a child to lose her mother, no matter how old she gets, as long as there is a true love between them. Germaine suffered a lot of pain the last few years of her life, and the quality of her life had become horrendously dismal, so it is best for her that she is now at peace at last. I will always feel her good influence on myself in my life. When I am interviewed on TV, I shall hear her voice in the back of my mind saying, "Wear a brassiere, please" and "Don't say stupid banal things you might regret afterward."

I am now *child no more*, and yet my mother's presence will always be with me. Your loving daughter, Veraatje.

Acknowledgments

I want to thank my dear friend Eric Kohn for his patience in painstakingly putting together the pieces of this jigsaw puzzle with me. He helped me to assemble these intertwined narratives and impressions into a coherent story—my story.

Furthermore, I want to thank Hetty, who looked after Germaine for so many years, and Pauline, another dear friend, for producing the lovely booklets with my eulogy and some beautiful German poetry for my mother's funeral.

And of course thanks to my lovers, Dia and Romke, who stood beside me during the most difficult days of my life. I wish to express my gratitude to this lovely and ever-growing X Team, a group of creative, faithful, and loyal friends. They supported me through the agony of those last days, and the painful aftermath, and assisted me in the production of many theater performances in my house. They read many chapters of this book in draft and gave me their wholehearted support in this project.

Last but not least, my thanks to James and Christopher, who have shared my house with me over the years, looking after my daily needs—food, drink, my dogs, entertainment—and imposing order out of chaos in my house and in my life.

Visit Xaviera at www.xavierahollander.com, or E-mail her at xaviera@xavierahollander.com.